ASSESSMENT IN SPORT PSYCHOLOGY

Assessment in Sport Psychology

Robert M. Nideffer and Marc-Simon Sagal

Fitness Information Technology, Inc.

•

P.O. Box 4425

•

Morgantown, WV 26504-4425

Library of Congress Card Catalog Number: 01-130179

ISBN: 1-885693-28-1

Copyeditor: Candace Jordan
Cover Design: Michael Komarck
Managing Editor: Geoffrey C. Fuller
Production Editor: Craig Hines
Proofreader: Candace Jordan
Indexer: Maria denBoer
Printed by Data Reproductions, Inc.

10 9 8 7 6 5 4 3 2 1

Fitness Information Technology, Inc.
P.O. Box 4425, University Avenue
Morgantown, WV 26504 USA
800.477.4348
304.599.3483 phone
304.599.3482 fax
Email: fit@fitinfotech.com
Website: www.fitinfotech.com

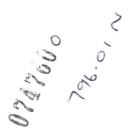

Dedicated to Ros, Jeffrey, and Jason. Special thanks to Dennis Selder at SDSU, Len Zaichkowsky at BU, Keith Henschen at the University of Utah, Jeff Bond and the Australian Institute for Sport, and to Alberto Cei and Umberto Manili at the Scuola dello Sport in Rome for their continued encouragement and support.

—Robert Nideffer

To my parents, Paul and Karen, and my wife, Courtney, for their love and support. A special thanks to my father for all his help and for giving me my first book on sport psychology.

—Marc Sagal

Contents

Preface

- Will this person put it all together when everything is on the line?

- Are certain conditions more likely to lead to success or failure for this individual?

- Will this person be able to fit in and become an effective, contributing member of this team?

- What steps can be taken to make sure this individual gets the very best out of him- or herself when it really counts?

- Will this person be able, and willing, to make the changes required to be more successful?

These are important questions. Questions that often take months to answer. Questions that in today's highly competitive environment often spell the difference between success and failure, not only for individuals, but also for entire teams and organizations. At the upper levels of performance, in situations where competing individuals and teams have all the technical skill and tactical knowledge required to be successful, psychological factors become the most important determinants of outcome. The ability to control emotions, to communicate effectively, and to perform under pressure is what separates winners from losers. This ability is equally important during skill acquisition. At such times it is the coach or team leader's abilities, however, that dictate whether learning will take place, or whether the experience will motivate the individual to continue to develop.

If you could shorten the length of time it takes to answer questions like those listed above by 6 months to a year, would it make a difference to the people you work with? We can do a better job of answering these types of questions, with nothing more than psychological test information and a one-hour interview, than most coaches or managers can after working with the individual on a daily basis for 6 months. More often than not, feedback of test information results in such comments as

- *I can't believe you got all that from a test.*

- *Have you been at my practices and games for the past year?*

- *That's exactly what happened yesterday.*

- *That's amazing, you described the situation perfectly.*

- *Can you imagine where we could be if we'd known this stuff 3 years ago?*

In spite of the impact psychological assessment can have on success, formal testing rarely takes place. With so much to gain, why aren't more professionals using information from psychological inventories to help them validate and improve the quality of the services they provide? Within the field of psychology in general, and sport psychology in particular, there are several reasons for what can best be described as an antitesting bias.

Prior to the development of the professional schools in psychology in the late 1970s, the dominant training model in clinical psychology was referred to as *the Boulder model*, after a conference on training in clinical psychology held in Boulder, Colorado. Individuals educated under the Boulder model were trained as both practitioners and researchers. Within this model, psychological assessment provided the bridge between the art (application) and the science (research) of psychology. The goal of the Boulder model was to train individuals to function in both arenas. As researchers, they would be sensitive to applied issues. As practitioners, they would be sensitive to the need to validate and evaluate the services they provided. Most of the individuals who were trained under this model, however, either because of their own choosing or because of the demands of their jobs, moved strongly in one direction or the other.

The Boulder model, like all training models, had its strengths and weaknesses. Most of the individuals who were trained under that model became either scientists or practitioners. The science of psychology and the art of psychology seemed to be at odds. Most people attempted to resolve the apparent conflict by taking one side or the other. Few people, it seemed, were well suited to functioning in both worlds.

As time passed, the Boulder model became more focused on the science of psychology. Those students and faculty interested in applied activities became increasingly unhappy. Their discontent led to the development of professional schools with strong applied focus. The development of these schools widened the schism between scientist and practitioner. The assessment bridge became less important to both sides, and the quantity and quality of training in assessment decreased.

Today, most faculty in sport psychology programs have had little or no formal training in psychological assessment. In addition, they have been exposed to a research literature with a fairly strong antitesting bias. Prior to the 1970s, most of the psychological inventories used in the field of sport psychology had been developed to help understand and to diagnose mental illness. Serious problems arose when inventories designed to measure pathology were used to assess healthy athletes. The items on these inventories lacked *face validity*, a deficiency that made it difficult for coaches and athletes to accept the testing process. Those individuals qualified to use the inventories tended to analyze the results within the context of the theory underlying each test. This caused the analysts to see performance problems as pathological and to apply clinical labels to athletes. Because the items on these inventories were not directly related to performance, the inventories had little predictive value. Small wonder that many individuals in the field became alienated from and biased against the use of psychological tests.

Changes have begun, but the process is surprisingly slow. Professional associations still tend to be either research oriented or application oriented. The stigma associated with the use of tests designed to measure psychopathology remains. Faculty who have had little or no formal training or experience in psychological assessment are understandably uncomfortable about teaching courses on the subject.

We are confident that assessment will become an increasingly important part of graduate education in sport psychology. The reason is simple: Sport has become big business. In today's highly competitive sports markets, much is at stake, and winning is what it's all about.

In the 1970s, we began to see the technical and tactical leveling of the playing field as Eastern European countries began to spend more money on the development of their athletes. As the rewards for winning grow, and as technical and tactical abilities equalize, psychological factors will play an increasingly significant role in determining success or failure. This makes the assessment of psychological talent crucial. Coaches, managers, owners, and the athletes themselves want to know if they have what it takes, psychologically as well as physically. Individuals are becoming more invested in identifying and developing their psychological skills.

Sport psychologists are beginning to uncover the links between thought processes and physiology and, as a result, are developing tools that have much greater utility and relevance. Interest in assessment and testing will continue to grow as researchers develop more sophisticated nonclinical tools. Changes in technology have made it easier to collect and to analyze information. Sport psychologists can now collaborate on research projects with individuals worldwide; consequently, they can increase sample sizes and design more complex studies. The resulting knowledge is power, not just for the sport psychologist but for the coach and athlete as well.

Today, more than ever before, sport psychology professionals must have the skills necessary to bridge the worlds of application and science. Sport psychology professionals are gaining credibility and have valuable services to offer. Their future depends on their relevance and on their ability to advance the science of their field. This book is our attempt to reintroduce the importance of assessment as a bridge between the art and the science of the services we provide as sport psychology professionals. Our goal is to give students and instructors a practical guide they can use to

- more accurately evaluate the contributions that psychological tests can make to applied research and service provision;

- become more sensitive to the ethical issues associated with the use of psychological tests in research and in service provision;

- begin to develop the interviewing and interpretive skills necessary to ask the right questions, to consensually validate test results and conclusions, and to provide powerful feedback to the client for team building, screening, selection, and performance enhancement, and

- gain an appreciation for the ways in which advancing technologies can enhance the ability to accurately assess human behavior.

This is not a book about tests and measurements. We have made no attempt to review or to pass judgment on various psychological tests. We believe that the evaluation of a psychological inventory must be made by the individual using the test, within the context of his or her particular performance arena. This book uses the Theory of Attentional and Interpersonal Style as a template to highlight critical issues in assessment. The theory also provides instructors and students with a conceptual framework they can use to begin evaluating the assessment and performance intervention processes.

Clearly, we believe that the Theory of Attentional and Interpersonal Style is valuable to both researchers and practitioners. This isn't to say the theory is without problems. Indeed, some of these problems will be presented as part of our effort to highlight fundamental issues. Other theories or instruments may prove to be as useful. The choice of framework is ultimately a decision that you must make. Our goal, here, is to provide you with the necessary tools to make these judgments in an informed, logical, and practical way.[1]

[1.] Throughout this text, when both authors speak with a common voice, we have used "we." Whenever "I" is used, the speaker is the first author (Robert Nideffer).

Testing and the Assessment Process 1

Human beings are constantly engaged in the process of assessment. In order to understand, predict, and control themselves and their world, people must be able to evaluate and to assess. They assess traffic conditions and the behaviors of drivers before crossing the street. They assess the physical and mental skills and abilities of those they work with and compete against. They assess moods, attitudes, and interests. They assess their own physical, mental, and emotional states prior to major competitions and other big events. The list is endless.

Testing in general, and psychological testing in particular, is just one part of a larger assessment process. Is testing necessary? Aren't the decisions you make good enough without it? Will testing really add anything significant to what you already know? We believe psychological tests should play an important role in the larger assessment process. It is absolutely critical, however, that you realize testing is not a substitute for the assessment process. To assume this would be like assuming that you only need one ingredient to bake a cake.

Assessment aims at enhancing your ability to understand, predict, and control behavior. To accomplish this objective, you must first accumulate relevant data. Typically, the data that go into the day-to-day assessment recipe include past history, behavioral observations, interview information, and opinions of others.

Once the information has been gathered, it must be evaluated. Dumping all of the ingredients into a pan doesn't give you a cake. Likewise, the simple accumulation of information or data doesn't automatically lead to the right conclusions or decisions. The ingredients need to be blended. If the cake ingredients don't blend well (e.g., the oil separates, the flour is too lumpy), your cake will turn out poorly. The data that go into the assessment process also must be blended. Blending, in this case, is a process we call *consensual validation*. The information is examined for reliability and consistency. In other words, does the information from one source support the information from another?

Finally, based on how well the different parts fit together, you must make a prediction about the quality of the end product. How good will the cake be? How accurate will your prediction be? If you are confident, you behave in a manner consistent with the anticipated outcome. The baker who has used the same recipe a dozen times, and who has had it come out well every time, isn't afraid to serve the cake to a group of gourmets. The service provider who has had the same data in the past indicate a particular type of performance problem will be confident enough to take steps to eliminate or at least to minimize that problem before it occurs.

To have accomplished what you have already accomplished in your life, you must be fairly good at assessing the world around you. You've achieved a certain level of proficiency without using psychological tests, so why use them? We look at it this way: If there is room for improvement in your ability to understand, predict, and control yourself and the world around you, then the use of psychological testing may be comparable to the icing on your cake.

In this chapter, we will present some of the ways psychological inventories or tests can be used to reduce mistakes and to enhance the quality of services professional consultants provide to their clients. As you read on, be sure to engage in the assessment process yourself. Evaluate the accuracy of what we say relative to your own experiences. Be critical of us and of yourself. Once you've evaluated what we have presented, take the time to gather additional data by discussing the issues with colleagues, instructors, and classmates. Then draw your own conclusions.

Many of you may believe that we should not use psychological tests because responses are subjective (reflective more of individual beliefs and opinions than of actual behavior). We strongly disagree. It is precisely this subjectivity that allows for insight into performance issues. In other words, you will often want to use certain tests because they are subjective. What do you suppose interferes most with an individual's ability to perform, to communicate, and to make appropriate changes in problem behaviors? We believe the answer is an inaccurate self-perception.

For example, Mike may see himself as the most talented individual on the team. Kate may see Mike as arrogant, pompous, and totally out of touch with reality. The discrepancy in perception leads to interpersonal conflict. Misperceptions lead to additional problems. When people chronically underestimate their abilities, they underachieve. If you see me as impulsive and emotionally out of control but I don't see myself that way, there is little chance that I'll change my behavior, even if it is causing me to fail.

When an individual responds to a psychological test, that person is describing him- or herself to you. The resulting behavioral template can then be compared with past performance and with observations made by you and by others. You learn more and have more to offer when you find discrepancies between an individual's self-perceptions and the perceptions others have of that person.

People use their past experiences to develop a way of viewing the world. They see what they are prepared to see. When coaches evaluate an athlete's performance, they tend to assess technical and tactical skills. When general managers evaluate coaches or potential team members, they pay serious attention to communication skills and to the ability to fit in with the other members of the organization. What people assess and how they assess are determined by their past experience and by the unique requirements of different situations. Some are good at assessing and predicting success within very specific performance arenas but are less skilled at accurately evaluating others. A coach may be great at assessing physical talent but insensitive to interpersonal skills and abilities. A manager may be so focused on assessing an individual's ability to get along with others that he or she fails to adequately assess talent.

The use of psychological tests is one way to expand your worldview and your knowledge base. Tests express the worldview of their developer(s). The developer, on the basis of his or her experience, decides what to measure. Statistical procedures are then used to establish the reliability and validity of that measurement.

Why are some people much better than others at assessing people and situations? It is because they have a better sense of what to look for. They are also better at digesting, organizing, and consensually validating or invalidating the information they gather.

Have you noticed how some students are especially good at predicting what a professor is "looking for" on an exam? We certainly have. We see students all the time who know just what to study and just what to ignore. We also see students who work every bit as hard, if not harder, and who learn just as much, if not more, but who do not receive the same good grades. These less proficient assessors have not learned how to get the high marks. You could say they have learned the wrong things.

Students who are good at assessing the professor's expectations can efficiently separate *signal* from *noise*. Their experience with other professors, like the experience of a seasoned athlete, has taught them what to attend to and what to ignore. If these students took the time to think critically about what it is that tells them what to study, they could teach it to others and perhaps even provide others with a tool to measure it. An experienced defensive lineman in football has learned to ignore the cadence of the signal caller and to pay attention to the movement of the ball. The inexperienced or anxious lineman attends to the cadence and is drawn offside. Learning what to attend to is critical. An inventory can help you do this.

When you consider using a test or inventory, ask yourself the following questions:

- Was the developer of the inventory skilled at assessing the kinds of behaviors you want to assess?

- Was he or she interested in drawing the same kinds of conclusions and making the same kinds of decisions that interest you?

- Are there others who are good at making the kind of predictions you want to make, who attribute some of their success to the kind of information provided by the inventory?

- Does the inventory add to your ability to identify and measure behaviors that are relevant to drawing conclusions about the issues you face?

Testing Saves Time

What are some of the reasons so many marriages end in divorce? First, the newness and excitement of marriage often keep couples focused on the positives. Although negative indicators relative to sustaining a lasting relationship are present, they are ignored or overlooked. Second, some problems take a while to develop, and occur within situational contexts. Months or years may pass before the situation that triggers the problem occurs. An individual may be prone to extramarital affairs, for example, but may have little or no opportunity to wander.

If we interview someone for a job, we may or may not ask all of the pertinent questions. Like most people, even if we have a structured interview or agenda, we're going to get sidetracked from time to time. If we observe the individual's performance, will we see it under enough different circumstances to be able to generalize from what we see to new situations? Selecting instruments that measure a broad range of performance-relevant variables, and structuring the assessment situation so that you have an opportunity to observe the behavior of the individual under different levels of arousal, can dramatically shorten the length of time it takes to zero in on critical issues. The following is a case in point.

John was a college sophomore who had been running track for 2 years. He had tremendous speed and was a member of a world-record-holding relay team. His coach saw him as the perfect athlete. He worked incredibly hard and never questioned what he was asked to do. The coach never heard him complain, and when John was asked for his feelings on an issue, he always had something positive to say. His coach believed in the importance of psychological and physical skills. We were brought in to assess the team and to provide members with feedback so they could hone their mental skills. (Keep in mind that the coach didn't see any major problems. He believed that the psychological and physical skills of his athletes were quite good but that there was room for improvement.)

Neither John's past performances nor his day-to-day behavior, as described by the coach, provided any indication of a psychological or emotional problem. We expected to find an effective-looking test profile, but we were very wrong. Frankly, when we saw how John had responded to the inventory, we were shocked.

Not everything was surprising: Consistent with the coach's description, John's test results indicated he saw himself as extremely focused and dedicated. He described himself as a hard worker and very competitive. But his scores also indicated that he was quiet, and even less likely to speak out when he became angry. On the rare occasions that he would speak up, he tended to say something positive and supportive. Indeed, with respect to outward behavior, there was no disagreement between what the coach saw, what we saw, and what the test indicated. No one on the outside had any idea about what was really happening inside John's head.

John's test results also indicated that he was anxious and depressed. His ability to concentrate effectively was impaired by all the rumination and worry. He was easily distracted, and his self-confidence was low. John's extreme introversion (again as indicated by testing), combined with his reluctance to express thoughts, ideas, anger, and dissatisfaction, prevented people from knowing what was really going on. He had been the coach's best performer for 2 years, but the coach didn't really know him at all, nor, apparently, did anyone else. Testing had given John an opportunity to express himself, a chance to let someone know about his internal struggle.

Talking with John wasn't easy, because he had to be drawn out, but once he felt comfortable, the issue(s) became clear. John was a Black athlete from a very close family and he was running track for a White coach at a predominantly White university in the South. Making friends was not easy for him. Because he lacked confidence in his intellectual skills, he would not speak out for fear of looking foolish. He believed that only his athletic ability had secured his admission into school. In his mind, he passed courses not because he had earned a passing grade (even though he had) but because he was an athlete. Many of his fears were directly and indirectly reinforced by his surroundings.

John was ready to leave the university and had been talking to a Black coach from a college near his home about transferring. It would have been a poor decision, both from an academic and from a sport perspective. He was unlikely to get the same level of competition and exposure at the other school. Fortunately, the coach he had approached realized this and told John that while he would love to have him on the team, he wanted John to have a serious talk with his current coach before making any decision.

Once John's coach saw what was troubling his star athlete, it was not hard to turn things around. The coach truly cared about John. He was willing to listen and was able to understand. He stopped interpreting John's silence as an indication that everything was great. He made it a point to spend time one-on-one with John and to talk about how things were going, away from the track. He took more of an interest in John's academic work and helped him to realize that he really was performing well, both on and off the track. Other Black athletes on the team had been similarly unaware of John's feelings. The coach enlisted some of the athletes he knew well to work on getting to know John better. The coach's efforts paid off for everyone: John graduated 2 years later, and the relay team he was on set a world record.

Testing Contributes to Fairness in the Evaluation Process

Many people argue that psychological tests should not be used for making selection and screening decisions. They point out that correlations indicating the predictive validity of the inventories are too low. Because the decisions being made (e.g., selecting an Olympic team or drafting a player in the first round) are so important, and because tests are far from perfect predictors of performance, there is great reluctance to use them. We agree, but only in part. While tests alone should not be used to make selection and screening decisions, they should be a part of the decision-making process. Tests don't make decisions; people do. Individuals who rely on tests to make the decisions for them (by creating absolute cutoff scores) are behaving unethically.

On the other hand, structured psychological testing adds an element of fairness to the evaluation process because it provides an equal opportunity for those being tested to show evidence of certain behaviors and to perform in similar ways. While it is true that responses and attitudes toward the testing process may not be the same (for cultural, educational, and genetic reasons, etc.), this applies to almost all aspects of the assessment process, including interviews. For this reason, you should never rely on one set of data, whether those data come from testing, from an interview, from a resumé, or from behavioral observations. Instead, gather information from a variety of methods and then compare the information in order to consensually validate your conclusions (Garb, 1998).

The Process of Testing Improves Performance

We use tests because we believe the resulting information will be accurate and useful in developing programs for performance enhancement. At times, however, the testing process and the information provided by tests can be useful even if the information is inaccurate or irrelevant. This is often the case when an individual's anxiety level is high and when what that person needs more than anything else is simple structure and direction to help control the anxiety. With highly anxious individuals, any answer, within reason, can provide enough structure to reduce anxiety and return performance to normal. Here's an example:

Frank was attempting to make the Olympic team in the sport of international skeet shooting. Although an excellent shot, he knew he wasn't of the caliber to make the team. He was happy to be skilled enough to participate in the trials. Frank was extremely bright and a good assessor of his, and others', abilities. On the morning of the first day of the trials, Frank was practicing with Jeff. Frank knew Jeff was far and away the best shot at the trials, and he had been a fan of Jeff's for years. In fact, he had modeled his shooting after Jeff's. As he watched Jeff perform, Frank sensed that Jeff was anxious. As the practice session continued, Jeff's agitation became more apparent; he started talking to himself, complaining about the way he was hitting targets. Frank, watching his friend shoot, couldn't identify any problems. Jeff seemed to be "pounding" the targets; he wasn't missing a thing. Yet Frank could tell that if Jeff's frustration continued, Jeff would soon tighten up enough to start missing targets. It wouldn't take more than 4 missed targets out of 200 to keep Jeff from making the team.

Frank knew he wasn't going to make the team, and he really wanted his country to do well. He wanted Jeff on the team. To Frank's surprise, Jeff turned to him and asked him what was wrong. For a moment, Frank was at a loss for words. Here was one of the best shots in the world—a person Frank looked to for insight and instruction—asking for help. Fortunately, Frank was smart enough to realize that the worst thing to do when an individual is losing confidence is to encourage the person to make a significant change in any of the strategies that have succeeded in the past. Having observed Jeff's shooting, Frank couldn't detect any problems, yet he knew that telling Jeff there was nothing wrong wouldn't help matters. Since Jeff believed there was a problem, saying that everything looked fine might even make matters worse. Frank felt trapped. To offer a suggestion that would change Jeff's shooting would be more likely to hurt than to help. To say that he couldn't see anything wrong wouldn't bring Jeff's confidence back.

But Frank was savvy. After a moment's thought, he looked Jeff in the eye and said, "You know, I did notice something that you seem to be doing differently. It seems to me that in the past you've had your left foot turned about a half-inch more, toward the left." Frank had not really noticed this, but he knew that he was telling Jeff to do something that would not affect his shooting one way or the other. However, it would give Jeff something to think about besides his anxiety. It would provide an explanation for the problem and give Jeff something to do about it.

Jeff responded to Frank's suggestion, and his anxiety decreased. To Frank, there was no visible change in the way Jeff was hitting targets, but Jeff was satisfied and "back in the zone." Jeff made the team without any problems.

The feeling that something is wrong, or that something may go wrong, can destroy the performance of even highly skilled individuals. Ambiguity and uncertainty generate mental distractions and physiological changes that can destroy performance. Sometimes even bad news can be better than no news at all. A patient who fears she is ill may be somewhat relieved when she finds out she actually is. Knowing what the problem is provides structure and direction; it gives the individual involved a chance to regain a sense of control and an opportunity to start fixing things.

Information from psychological tests can be used to provide individuals with structure and direction. It some cases, particularly when dealing with anxiety and fear of failure, the accuracy of the explanation may not matter. Providing increased structure and guidance based on test data, or on anything else, can help as long as execution is not affected in the process. The only problem with this approach is that you haven't gotten to the root of the anxiety and self-doubt. Your solution will only be temporary. Are you thinking that the "active ingredient" in this type of intervention is more like a placebo than it is real medicine? This is certainly something interesting to contemplate.

We would almost never suggest that you use a test solely to provide structure. Most of the performance problems we encounter are complicated and worsened by anxiety and a lack of self-confidence. Structure can often improve performance by reducing anxiety and increasing confidence, but your ultimate goal is to find the root cause and resolve the problem. Ideally, testing will help you do all of these things.

Self-confidence can be very traitlike. Many of you are probably confident in your ability to do tasks in a variety of performance arenas. No matter how confident you are, however, there will be times when that confidence disappears. When it does, especially for individuals who are highly confident in most situations, it can be difficult to recover. People who have frequent losses of faith or confidence in themselves find it easy to turn to others for structure and direction. But if you are highly confident, if you take pride in solving your own problems, and if you believe that you know yourself better than anyone else does, whom do you trust and to whom do you turn when the wheels come off? Looking to others for help and structure can be especially hard for confident coaches and athletes.

Surprisingly, it is sometimes easier for highly confident individuals to trust the information they obtain from psychological inventories than it is for them to trust their own ideas or the opinions of others—never mind that the feedback they receive from tests reflects their own thoughts and feelings. Somehow, they see test results as more objective and feel less threatened by the results. They feel they have to know as much as other people, but they don't feel they have to know as much as the test. When this happens, test results can have very powerful calming and motivating effects, as long as they are interpreted in a way that yields understanding and direction.

The structure and direction obtained through test results can be equally valuable to the professional. We don't usually have ready-made answers to the myriad problems that bring people to us. We form tentative hypotheses and have more or less faith in these hypotheses depending on the information we have been able to gather. If we don't have confidence in our understanding of the issues, we can't provide the structure and the direction the client needs. When test results confirm our hypotheses, our confidence is increased, and this comes across to the client.

We would like to ask you to think critically about what you've read up to this point. Think about these questions and, if you are so inclined, discuss them with others:

- Do you agree that testing can be used to help refine your evaluation process by giving you information you might otherwise have overlooked?

- If you agree that the experts who develop tests have something to teach you that will make you better at understanding, predicting, and controlling behavior, then once you understand the theory behind the test, why would you still need the test itself?

- Do you understand how important a belief in knowing where you are going is to successful performance? Why is it so important?

- If test results are invalid, but the structure and direction the results provide improve performance, is there any difference between this process and a doctor's administration of a placebo to relieve pain?

- Would using tests as placebos raise any ethical concerns for you?

Earlier, we suggested that one reason some people are better at assessing and at accurately predicting behavior is that they are better at digesting, organizing, and consensually validating or invalidating information from tests and other sources. Before closing this chapter, we would like to discuss this in more detail.

Two people can be given the same information but draw very different conclusions. Seasoning and experience play a major role in the integration of information. You may know what each piece of information means when you view it in isolation, but putting the pieces together can take you to a new level. The ability to combine elements and to take isolated pieces of information from test scores, behavioral observations, past history, and interviews is critical. The skill to consensually validate information and to anticipate and predict the consequences of future interactions is something you can and must develop.

Developing your interpretive skills is a topic we will deal with throughout the book. To improve, you must constantly ask yourself to critically evaluate issues and information. This is just a practical application of the *scientific method*. Form hypotheses and test them out. When you ask a question like "Will the use of tests improve my ability to provide services to others?" this question leads to a prediction or hypothesis: "Yes, it will," or "No, it won't." Force yourself to identify, critically examine, and test the bits of data that brought about your hypothesis, then draw conclusions and refine your original assumption.

Throughout this book, we will provide you with questions and will ask you to generate and test hypotheses. There is no shortcut to effective, psychologically oriented service provision, no magic formula. The best equipment and information available are as useless as a plane without a pilot if you cannot evaluate information critically and, when necessary, apply it to new situations.

Suggested Readings

Garb, H. N. (1998). *Studying the clinician.* Washington, DC: American Psychological Association.

Maloney, M. P., & Ward, M. P. (1976). *Psychological assessment: A conceptual approach.* New York: Oxford University Press.

What You Should Be Measuring 2

In chapter 1, we presented some of the reasons to consider using tests in the assessment process. In this chapter, we want to talk about what you should be trying to evaluate. Assessment should be driven by the particular problem you are trying to solve. The goal here, like the goal most service providers have in sport, organizational, and industrial psychology, is to help people optimize performance—to help them perform to potential.

People come to professionals for help because they feel as though they have failed to accomplish a desired goal and/or because they believe professionals can help them achieve their objectives. The client defines the issue, which may be as broad as helping an entire team work together or as narrow as improving the start of a downhill skier.

Whatever the problem, you must be ready to respond. To do so, you need to have a reasonable idea of what you should observe and measure; more importantly, you must know what areas to avoid. With this in mind, take some time here to ask yourself, and to discuss with others, the psychological characteristics you think would be important to measure if you were helping the following individuals or teams deal with these issues:

- a downhill skier who is recovering from an injury,

- an NFL coach who has problems communicating with his team,

- a youth-sport hockey player who becomes "too anxious,"

- a youth-sport coach who has a team that isn't performing,

- a diver who loses control of her anger and frustration,

- an NBA player who doesn't seem motivated, or

- a Major League Baseball pitcher who has control problems.

Before you read on, answer this: Did you think about the characteristics you would like to measure? If you did think about them, did you

- identify any characteristics you wanted to measure that were applicable to several of the identified problems? In other words, were the characteristics related to performance across a wide variety of situations and settings?

- identify characteristics that were unique to a particular issue or performance arena?

- draw any conclusions about the amount of technical and tactical knowledge about each sport you would need in order to be helpful?

Those who are new to the assessment world may feel overwhelmed by all of the information they think they ought to have. They often assume that they need a great deal of tactical and technical knowledge about each sport, and they may perceive a need to measure physical skills and abilities as well as psychological ones. Frequently, they behave as if they must have the knowledge of a coach, an exercise physiologist, a nutritionist, a counselor, and a sport consultant all rolled into one.

We would like to emphasize that there is a very large difference between what you *need* to know and what it would be *nice* to know. A major problem for athletes is "paralysis by analysis." The same is true for sport psychology consultants. We can help narrow your focus. In the next few pages, we will discuss what you do and do not need to know from technical, tactical, and clinical perspectives.

You Don't Have to Be a Coach

Leave the coaching of technical and tactical skills to the coaching staff. You don't have to have extensive knowledge of every sport to be helpful to an athlete. What you should have is a fan's appreciation of the sport and a working knowledge of the jargon.

Sometimes athletes will seek your help to accomplish a goal (e.g., to make an Olympic team). In such cases, you will need the ability to determine whether he or she has or can obtain the tactical or technical skills required to succeed; otherwise, you will be wasting your time and the athlete's. You don't, however, have to be a coach to do this. You can gather the necessary information simply by asking the athlete, by questioning a knowledgeable trainer or coach, and by looking at the athlete's history. You do require a general understanding of how thought processes interact with physiology to affect performance and decision-making skills. You must be able to provide the coach and the athlete with the links between thought processes, focus of concentration, and performance, and be capable of showing how thought processes can detrimentally affect concentration and physiology. In other words, you need the resources to explain exactly how thought processes affect the athlete's decision making, his or her technique, and the biomechanics of performance. It is important for you to understand how altering the athlete's focus of attention can lead to positive changes in decision making and in technique. Unless you are a coach or a biomechanist, you are not likely to know exactly how the athlete should be performing biomechanically or what the athlete should be attending to. This point is very important and underlies your need to work through the coach and the sport scientist.

Mental factors affect athletic performance. When you provide mental training or use a psychological technique like relaxation or imagery, your intervention will help only if it affects performance-relevant physiology and the speed and accuracy of decision making. To be credible, and to be sure you are not doing something that will hurt performance, you should know the technical and tactical keys to successful performance. This is where the coach comes in. Here is an example:

A sprinter knows she can run the 100 in 10.9 because she has done it before. The problem is that she has never run faster than 11.1 in a big race. She's preparing to compete in the Olympic trials and wants you to help her run 10.9. You should be asking the athlete and the coach, "What determines how quickly she reaches the finish line?" Try to get the simplest explanation you can, the one that zeros in on the physical parameters that determine success or failure. Suppose the responses are (a) speed out of the blocks, (b) speed of turnover (how many strides she takes within a specified period of time), and (c) stride length. To help the sprinter, you have to help her to optimize these three variables. How will your intervention do that? Which of the three variables will your intervention affect, and how? What do you know about the interaction between mental and physical processes that will convince the athlete and the coach that you can help?

The Mind-Body Connection

Sport competition provides a unique opportunity to view clearly the interaction between mind and body, to see the effects of pressure on performance and to experience the consequences. Observable physiological signs or behaviors indicate when an individual lacks sufficient mental or physical skill to be successful. Coaches and biomechanists are experts at identifying breakdowns in motor performance and technique. They can point these out to you quite easily. Remember that the identified problem behaviors may be due to either a lack of technical or a lack of psychological skill. You and the coach must agree on which of these is the root of the problem.

Jim is missing his volleys because he isn't focused appropriately on the ball. Sharon is double-faulting because her ball toss is too far out in front and not high enough. Ali is dropping the ball because he is getting distracted by the defender. These are the consequences of problems, the results, but knowing that a problem exists is not enough. It is essential that you see and understand the process and that you identify the cause of the problem. Each of the above problems might occur either because the individuals have not yet developed the physiological skill sets required to perform consistently or because increasing pressure has interfered with the their ability to execute the skills that they do have.

As a general rule, when athletes have repeatedly demonstrated the capacity to perform at the desired level, they have developed the necessary technical and tactical skills. Any problems that occur once those skill sets have been developed can probably be attributed to psychological variables, especially if the mistakes have a pattern—a pattern that shows a clear connection between the problem and situational factors we would normally expect to significantly increase or decrease the emotional importance of the competition or performance. On the other hand, when the athlete has not demonstrated the ability to consistently perform in the desired way, it is usually because physical, rather than psychological, skills require development (Nideffer, 1992).

Let's assume that your athlete has the necessary technical skills and tactical knowledge. Under these conditions, your understanding of the interaction between mental and physical processes is your own theory of human performance. Your theory should be able to explain how mental processes affect a sprinter's stride length, prevent a tennis player from getting down low for a volley, or cause a golfer to leave a critical putt a foot short of the hole. You need a theory that can explain how physiological processes can keep a receiver from attending to a ball, a sprinter from getting out of the starting blocks quickly enough, or a basketball player from seeing the open man. Your theory must help to clarify why some people perform well under pressure and others do not. Your understanding of this process is what will enable you to trace a problem from its consequences back to its root. How you see this process determines the line of questioning you will take in an interview and the types of instruments you will use when testing.

Human behavior is a very complex process. No theories provide a complete understanding. Some, like the Inverted-U, are relatively simple (Yerkes & Dodson, 1908); others, like psychoanalytic theory, are more complex (Freud, 1940). You need a theory that helps you to understand, predict, and control the relevant range of behaviors you encounter. The theoretical constructs that follow are the ones we use. They have helped us respond to the needs of high-level performers for the past 20 years, and they provide a compelling and useful explication of the process of performing. Using these theoretical constructs, we have convinced coaches and athletes to accept our psychological interventions. You should not feel limited by these constructs, however. In fact, we challenge you to improve upon them.

To understand human performance you must know something about what we call the *building blocks of performance*. You also require some knowledge of the connection between emotional arousal and these building blocks. Finally, you must understand the role self-confidence plays in recovery from mistakes and from the unexpected.

The Building Blocks of Performance

Most tests measure complex constructs like anxiety, intelligence, motivation, concentration, and empathy rather than measuring the building blocks of these complex constructs. To measure empathy, for example, questions are usually generated that have face validity and provide sound evidence of the presence or absence of the behavior: "Are you able to feel what others feel?" or "Are you able to put yourself in other people's shoes in order to better understand things from their point of view?" The subject's answers to these complex questions are calculated, and the final score on the inventory is assumed to measure empathy.

Information gathered this way is not very useful. If the individual's score on the empathy measure is low, the test hasn't helped us determine why. A low score provides no indication as to the specific steps that should be taken to improve. That psychologists develop tests in this way shouldn't be too surprising; after all, this is the way most of us evaluate people. If we want to know whether a person can swim, we put him or her in the pool and see what happens. If we want people to tell us whether they can swim, we ask a question like "Can you swim?" We may even ask them to qualify their answers with modifiers like "very well," "pretty good," "average," "not very well," "not at all." This enables us to learn something about people, yet it does not give us all the information we need in order to help them.

A good swimming coach doesn't just look to see if the person makes it to the other end of the pool. A good swimming coach looks for evidence of the building blocks of swimming. She notices how the person uses his arms and legs, how he breathes, the position of his hands in the water, and so on. When a good swimming coach wants an athlete to swim faster, she doesn't just say, "Swim faster." Instead, her analysis of the basic building blocks of the skill allows her to give explicit instruction: "Move your right hand in this way. . . ." Similarly, what differentiates a good swimming coach from a bad one is what differentiates a good psychologist (or psychological test) from a bad one. When giving instructions to an athlete, a sport psychologist dealing with the mental side of competition must be as explicit as a coach. If you claim an ability to help athletes concentrate, you'd better be able to define the building blocks of concentration. Screaming, "Concentrate!" does not help any more than screaming, "Swim faster!"

The Role of Concentration in Performance

No one can perform optimally without attending to task-relevant cues. To understand what is involved in paying attention, you need to know the following:

- Focus of concentration constantly shifts in response to changing performance demands. The ability to make appropriate shifts is one of the building blocks of concentration.

- The shifts in concentration or focus of attention occur along two intersecting dimensions, a dimension of width and a dimension of direction.

- At any given point in time, focus of concentration falls into one of the four quadrants shown in Figure 1. Each of the four types of concentration represents a basic building block of concentration.

Athletes use a *broad-external* focus of concentration to quickly assess and intuitively react (i.e., respond without conscious thought) to changing conditions. They use a *broad-internal* focus of concentration to analyze

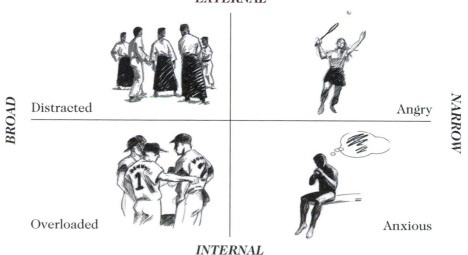

Figure 1. Mental Errors.

and plan. Past information is recalled and compared to present conditions in order to select and predict a course of action. A *narrow-internal* focus of concentration doesn't cut across time the way a broad-internal focus does; narrow-internal is a "here and now" way of attending. Athletes use it to mentally check how they are feeling and to systematize and mentally rehearse a performance. A *narrow-external* focus is used to minimize distractions and to focus energy in one direction in order to execute skills and to maximize effort (e.g., to swing at a pitch).

Concentration and Your Perception of the Passage of Time

To understand the relationship between your perception of the passage of time and your focus of concentration, think of your brain as a movie camera. Imagine that the camera is taking 40 pictures every second and that the camera moves in response to the changing demands of different performance settings.

For discussion purposes, imagine that as a general rule, the brain camera spends equal time aimed at each of the four concentration styles shown in Figure 1. Thus, in a 1-second period, the brain would take 10 pictures from a broad-external perspective, 10 pictures from a broad-internal perspective, 10 pictures from a narrow-external perspective, and 10 pictures from a narrow-internal perspective. Imagine, too, that this particular frequency of shifting is what you have learned to associate with the normal passage of time.

Continuing with this example, now imagine that you are a hitter in baseball. Envision that it takes 1 second for the ball to travel from the pitcher's hand to the plate. On a normal day, your brain will take 20 pictures of the ball as it approaches the plate (10 broad-external and 10 narrow-external). Your brain will use up the other 20 pictures planning (e.g., "It's a curve") and making adjustments in response to the movement of the ball (e.g., "Slow down the swing").

What happens when you "stay in the moment" or "get into the zone" is that your brain stops taking internal pictures. You go on automatic pilot; you have practiced hitting to the point that you don't need to consciously analyze your swing. Provided you have accurately determined the speed and trajectory of the pitch upon release, there is no need for conscious adjustments to your swing or your body position. Your brain stays focused externally for the entire second required for the ball to reach the plate, taking the optimal 40 pictures instead of just 20. Because you have focused exclusively on the ball for all 40 frames, time seems to slow down, and the ball appears to be coming toward you in slow motion.

The point we want you to remember here is that your perception of the passage of time depends on the frequency with which you shift concentration from an external focus to an internal one. The more you focus on the environment, the more slowly time seems to pass. The more you focus internally, the more quickly time seems to pass. You can relate to this when you think about what happens when you go to sleep and concentration is focused almost exclusively on internal processes. You can sleep for 8 hours but feel as if only minutes have passed.

Emotional Arousal and Focus of Concentration

Fluctuations in emotional arousal have a predictable effect on an individual's focus of attention and on the ability to shift back and forth between the different types of concentration. This relationship is reciprocal; an individual's focus of concentration can have a controlling effect on emotional arousal. An understanding of the relationship between attention and arousal, and of the conditions that impede a person's ability to control emotions and concentration, is critical in the design of effective intervention and training programs.

We are all familiar with the *fight-or-flight* response (Selye, 1974). Human beings are hardwired to respond to threatening situations with highly specific changes in both physiology and focus of concentration. These changes were built into the species to insure survival; but different people find different situations stressful, and this complicates our ability to understand, predict, and control behavior.

Choking

The following two factors, when present together, can generate emotional, physiological, and attentional disturbances that lead to the downward performance spiral often referred to as *choking*:

1. an individual who is in a situation where he or she is highly motivated to do well (it doesn't matter if the high level of motivation comes from a desire to make money, to please parents or the audience, to accomplish a lifetime goal, or to keep from dying), and

2. feedback that indicates things are not progressing as the individual would like.

Figure 2 shows what happens physically and mentally when an individual becomes stressed in a performance situation. Physiologically, several changes can have a detrimental effect on performance, especially performance that requires fine-motor coordination and timing. These changes include increases in respiration rate, heart rate, and muscle tension. Changes in muscle tension can interfere with athletic performance by causing early fatigue or cramps. They can alter body position and make it more difficult for an athlete to move and react: Sprinters and downhill skiers straighten up too much and lose speed; tennis players don't get low enough to adequately control their racquet faces when trying to volley. Finally, these

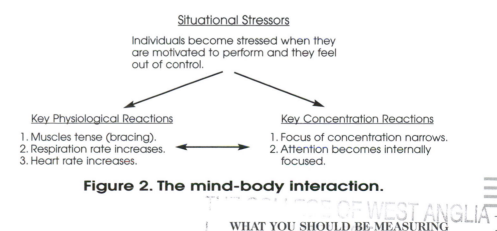

Figure 2. The mind-body interaction.

changes can affect fine-motor coordination and interfere with the athlete's sensitivity to critical kinesthetic feedback.

Changes in breathing can affect rhythm and timing. When athletes perform well, breathing is coordinated with movement and effort. There are times when it is appropriate to inhale and times when it is not. If you've ever been anxious when giving a speech, you know what we're talking about. People who are anxious when speaking in front of others often find themselves running out of air and breathing in the middle of sentences. They feel awkward, and this gets communicated to the audience. Athletes can run out of air the same way. They find themselves inhaling when they should be exhaling and vice versa.

In terms of the effects on concentration, increasing arousal causes attention to narrow. It's a built-in part of the fight-or-flight response. In a stressful situation, people focus so they can deal with the threat. This narrowing of attention results in a decreased awareness of peripheral cues. If the lost cues happen to be performance-relevant, it's a problem (Bacon, 1974; Easterbrook, 1959).

The next thing that happens to concentration under stressful conditions is that it begins to become more internally focused. Physiological changes occurring with increases in arousal are intense enough to direct focus of concentration inward (e.g., the athlete becomes conscious of his or her breathing or heart rate). When this happens, the athlete begins to feel rushed because time appears to speed up. The brain is taking more internal pictures (noise) and correspondingly fewer external pictures (signal). At this point, self-confidence, or faith in something, becomes absolutely critical to the athlete's ability to recover and to get back on task.

As disruptive as these changes in arousal can be, if the athlete has previously experienced them in the same situation and has been able to work his or her way out of trouble, the athlete will probably recover and perform successfully. For example, athletes with a history of success in demanding performance situations will likely be able to quickly remind themselves of this fact and use the comfort that comes from past success to relax and to refocus concentration on the task at hand. Confidence gained from past performance allows for quick recovery. Athletes who lack experience and are less able to focus attention effectively will have many more problems coping with pressure.

Choking occurs when confidence is low and when feedback (e.g., physiological change) is interpreted in negative or self-destructive ways. Anxiety from feeling out of control and rushed (as if time is speeding up) leads to further increases in emotional arousal and to a more narrow-internal focus of concentration. This creates a negative feedback loop between physical and mental processes, and all hope of performing successfully disappears. At this point, the athlete is incapable of acting as the instrument of his or her own recovery. A coach or teammate can call time-out and provide enough structure and direction for recovery to occur, but the athlete won't be able to do it alone.

As we said earlier, you don't need to have all of the technical and tactical knowledge and skill of a coach to work effectively with an athlete. However, you must have the skill to see the types of mistakes that are being made;

Table 1. Mental and Physical Links to Performance Errors

Problem	Explanation
A tennis player consistently double-faults on big points by hitting the ball into the net.	Negative thoughts lead to increased tension in neck and shoulders. This tension causes the ball toss to be lower and more in front. Anxiety and a narrow-internal focus of attention cause the player to feel rushed. As a result, she ducks her head, not watching the ball, and hits the ball into the net.
A 200-meter butterflyer swims his best times in practice meets and tightens up in the last 50 meters, when it counts.	
A golfer leaves big putts short.	
A gifted shortstop suddenly can't seem to hold on to the ball.	
A quarterback can't find his secondary receivers.	

you must understand and explain how the interaction between thought processes and emotional arousal, as we have presented them here, results in the performance difficulties that coaches and athletes present to you.

To test yourself, see if you can use the material just presented to analyze the problems listed in Table 1; then, identify some problems of your own and see how well the theoretical framework helps you to interpret them.

Clinical Issues

Unless you are trained as a clinical psychologist, psychiatrist, or psychiatric social worker, you should avoid working with problems that require in-depth counseling. The performance-relevant theory that educational sport psychologists and most organizational psychologists follow assumes that the individuals with whom they work are "normal"—normal in the sense that they don't have deep-seated, underlying emotional conflicts that prevent them from responding appropriately to training.

Staying away from clinical issues means staying away from tests designed to gather information about underlying emotional issues or conflicts that may well be at the root of an individual's problem. You should not employ projective tests like the Rorschach or diagnostic instruments like the MMPI. You are not in the business of testing or assessing unconscious conflicts or clinical pathology. You do, however, have to recognize clinical issues when they appear. An important question to ask yourself, and to find an answer to, is "When does a normal emotional issue become a clinical one?" (For more information on recognizing clinical issues, see the suggested readings at the end of this chapter.)

An athlete breaks up with a boyfriend or girlfriend. That breakup may have a negative impact on performance, but is this a clinical issue? A family member or friend dies, and again performance suffers, but is this a clinical issue? In both instances, the answer is "probably not." Certainly at the outset we wouldn't treat an individual's anxious or depressed responses to major life changes as clinical issues. Unless the person is unable to work through them in a normal, orderly way, we treat crises as a normal part of life. When we see that the individual is struggling—that the anxiety, depression, or anger is intensifying over time—it then becomes important for us to make a referral.

We expect people to think and behave in logical and rational ways. When athletes know what they need to do and appear to be highly motivated, yet continually act in ways that are self-destructive, a referral should be made to a clinically trained individual. When the emotions you see are irrational and an individual is unable to benefit from your support, direction, and structure, you need to make a referral. (It's at these times that a clinically trained individual might elect to administer tests such as the MMPI and Rorschach.)

Identifying Stressors

Our ultimate objective is to maximize performance across a wide range of performance settings. To do this, we must have enough technical and tactical knowledge in an area to recognize the kinds of mistakes being made. We require an understanding of the psychological (cognitive, intrapersonal, and interpersonal) processes that contribute to those mistakes.

Unless we understand the conditions that result in an individual's loss of concentration and inappropriate level of arousal, we cannot prevent problems. Unless we determine the building blocks of constructs like concentration and anxiety, we cannot identify what is causing the problems and thereby provide appropriate interventions. All we will be able to do is recognize and treat the symptoms of sub-par performance.

When an individual's mental and physical responses to a stressor interfere with performance, treat the problem as you would an illness. The general process by which the illness affects performance is similar for everyone. In every instance, the individual loses the ability to control concentration and emotional arousal. People differ, however, in terms of the types of situations that bring on the illness and in terms of the symptoms (types of mistakes) they manifest in response to the illness. Some athletes, for example, react with anger and frustration and behave in overly aggressive ways when they lose control (the *fight* response). Others react by becoming timid and tentative (the *flight* response). Then, too, there is the group that vacillates between the two responses, aggressive one minute and tentative the next.

It is naive to believe that once a person has learned to raise or lower arousal through the use of some technique within a particular situational context, he or she will be able to do the same in other situations. This kind of learning is not very generalizable. If it were, none of us would ever lose control, because we would have learned from those situations in which we were capable of controlling concentration and arousal. To be effective, interventions must be targeted. Because of the possible development of feedback loops that prevent recovery, interventions must sensitize the athlete to potential issues before they get out of control. This is where intrapersonal and interpersonal characteristics come into play.

Identifying Performance-Relevant, Traitlike Behaviors

Many personality characteristics are at least partially genetically determined. Even characteristics like extroversion, introversion, and optimism appear to have a genetic component. The presence of a genetic influence does not mean that behavior can't be modified or controlled by learning; the ability to effect change depends on how much of the behavior is *traitlike* (present across different situations) and how much of it is *situation-specific* (or *statelike*). Everyone differs with respect to how traitlike or statelike various performance-related behaviors are. One of the primary reasons for testing is to acquire a sense of the trans-situational stability (i.e., predictability) of critical behaviors. Again, the key question is, What are the critical factors we want to measure?

Psychologists have identified hundreds of personality characteristics, cognitive processes, attitudes, interpersonal behaviors, and needs. All of them may have some performance relevance at one time or another. Which ones are most important? Which factors are most likely to predict the conditions under which individuals will fail to adequately control concentration and emotional arousal? Which factors will be most useful in predicting whether or not the mistakes an individual makes are due to anxiety, tentativeness, anger, or overzealousness? What are the interpersonal and intrapersonal building blocks of performance?

In the next few pages, we will identify the cognitive abilities and interpersonal skills we believe to be the best predictors of behavior across performance situations. Before we do, however, give this topic some thought: Development of the ability to consistently perform near optimal levels in any situation is a long-term process. Assume someone has told you that a young golfer has all of the physical requirements necessary to become one of the best golfers in the world. Her parents and coach ask you, as the psychological expert, to help them anticipate where problems are likely to occur. They request your ongoing involvement to help prevent and overcome those problems.

What would you like to know about this young woman? What mental and interpersonal characteristics do you think she will need to succeed? Your willingness to take the time to identify the kinds of information you require is important. Remember, you are already making such predictions about people, whether or not you have explicitly identified the characteristics on which your predictions are based. By making those characteristics explicit, you will be more likely to effectively, and objectively, evaluate their role in performance. Table 2 provides a place for you to list the behaviors and characteristics you would like to know about.

If someone asked us to predict whether or not an Olympic-caliber athlete would be successful, we would probably start by identifying the cognitive behaviors and interpersonal characteristics that play an important role

Table 2. Mental and Interpersonal Skills Required for Success

	Mental skills	Interpersonal skills
	1.	1.
	2.	2.
	3.	3.
	4.	4.
	5.	5.
	6.	6.
	7.	7.
	8.	8.
	9.	9.
	10.	10.

in many different situations. The reason is simple: To win a gold medal in the Olympics, an athlete must perform well in various situations over an extended period of time. The athlete will often be tempted to give up or quit. Success depends on a great deal more than controlling concentration and arousal during a single event.

Performance-Relevant Cognitive Characteristics

Earlier in this chapter we described how the focus of concentration constantly moves along two intersecting axes, width and direction. In normal, day-to-day existence, everyone has the ability to shift focus of attention along these four dimensions. The concentration demands of different performance situations vary considerably. Many sport situations require very little conscious analysis; in fact, athletes seem to perform best when their focus of concentration is almost exclusively external (the "zone"). At these times, athletes rely primarily on instinct and on all the practice hours that have made necessary behaviors automatic.

In contrast to most sport situations, academic situations usually require an internal focus of concentration (e.g., analyzing, planning, problem solving, and theorizing). Although everyone seems capable of shifting from one focus to another, there are clear differences in terms of the willingness and ease with which individuals make these shifts.

Many highly effective researchers and academics are dominated by an internal focus of concentration. World-class athletes and technically oriented individuals have a predominantly narrow focus of concentration. Salespeople and charismatic leaders capitalize on their broad-external awareness in order to gauge how others are responding to them.

We want to know an individual's preferred or dominant concentration or attentional style. The more highly developed and traitlike one type of concentration is, relative to others, the more predictable the individual's behavior. The more dominant one style is, the easier it is to use it to identify situations in which the person will and will not perform well.

In addition to concentration skills, we want to know something about an individual's information-processing capacity. How busy and complex is that person's world? Some people are comfortable with, and very capable of dealing with, a number of different issues at the same time. They jump back and forth between tasks with relative ease and enjoy the challenge. In fact, they often grow bored and even anxious when things become routine. These people need change and new challenges. Others are more comfortable with structure and direction. They prefer to perform one task at a time. They don't like to be disturbed, and they become stressed and overloaded when they have to multitask.

When we examine the reasons people fail to accomplish goals and objectives, the importance of concentration skills and of the ability to shift from one focus to another in response to changing demands becomes obvious. An individual's greatest concentration strength can be, and often is, his or her Achilles' heel. Some people have had great success because of their sensitivity to the environment. When these people fail, it is often because their environmental awareness leads to distractions; they can't stay as focused (e.g., pros who are seduced by groupies and drugs). Other people achieve a relatively high level of performance because they are focused, but ultimately fail because they are too focused; they become inflexible and fail to adjust to new situations. Remember when Bjorn Borg insisted he would make a comeback in tennis using his old wooden racquet?

Individuals with great analytical skills can undermine themselves when they overanalyze and fail to stop thinking long enough to let themselves perform; the absentminded professor and the athlete suffering from "paralysis by analysis" are good examples. There are also those people who fail because they are too reactive, such as players who get ejected at critical times because they can't control their emotions enough to think about the consequences of a behavior.

To summarize, you will want to examine, from a cognitive standpoint, the individual's

- external awareness, or ability to read and react to the environment;

- ability to integrate information, to analyze, and to plan;

- ability to focus concentration (both to attend to details, thereby polishing and refining skills, and to avoid distraction under pressure);

- preference or need for change and diversity;

- tendency to become distracted by external/environmental cues;

- tendency to become overloaded with thoughts and feelings; and

- tendency to become too narrowly focused, unable to adjust to changing concentration requirements.

Performance-Relevant Interpersonal Skills (Personality Characteristics)

The extent to which human behavior is genetically and biologically determined and the extent to which it is learned are the subject of much debate. We will assume that both play an important role in the determination of who people are. From a practical standpoint, however, it doesn't really matter if a dominant behavior is a highly developed, learned habit or a natural response, because an individual can perform both automatically, without conscious direction or thought.

During the learning process, human beings constantly monitor and evaluate the effectiveness of their behavior and make adjustments in order to improve their level of performance. To modify highly practiced, automatic behaviors (the behaviors most athletes engage in during competition), however, athletes first must learn to inhibit what have become automatic responses. The key to this involves expanding personal awareness. This means becoming more sensitive to the behaviors they engage in automatically and being willing to modify those behaviors in order to adapt to situations calling for new responses.

Interpersonal behaviors, like concentration skills, can be traitlike for some individuals and situation-specific for others. In most instances, it is the traitlike behaviors that contribute most to success or failure. People experience success when the performance arena plays to their dominant concentration skills and interpersonal styles. They experience failure when the outcome of an important situation is in doubt, and their dominant concentration skills and interpersonal characteristics are not what the situation requires. Under such conditions, excessive arousal causes individuals to lose flexibility in their concentration and interpersonal skills; here, the same tools they use to build themselves up bring them down.

We use testing to sensitize people to their dominant behavior patterns and to show them how those patterns reduce their flexibility in high-pressure situations. Below, we describe the interpersonal characteristics that are relevant across situations.

Risk Taking

How conservative or conventional are you? How rigidly do you stick to the rules? How willing are you to bend the rules to accomplish objectives? Some coaches and athletes make it a point to do things their way. If the world doesn't like it, tough. They are stressed by, and rebel at, having to do things the way everyone else does. Others seem to need the structure and predictability that rules provide. These people stick closely to the rules and become agitated and stressed when a situation requires them to behave in an unconventional way or when others break the rules.

Control

To what extent are you willing to take responsibility for and control of not only your own behavior, but also of the behavior of others? To what extent does the performance situation place you in a leadership role? How important is it for you to function as a leader? As a follower?

Need for control is a traitlike characteristic for many people. Some individuals always want to be in the driver's seat; others are perfectly happy letting others make the decisions. The more extreme an individual is in either direction, the more that person will be stressed by situations that do not match his or her need. Individuals who want and need control become frustrated when they don't have it. Individuals who avoid taking a leadership role grow stressed when the situation forces that role upon them.

Confidence

How confident are you? How strong is your belief in your ability to master different situations? Some individuals always appear confident. Under pressure, overly confident people make such mistakes as failing to recognize weaknesses, disregarding criticism, and taking on responsibilities before they are ready. Individuals who lack confidence often make mistakes because they don't take necessary risks, don't take on leadership roles when they should, and don't set high enough goals.

Competitiveness

How competitive are you? Are you willing to go head to head with the competition? Some people have to beat everyone they encounter, no matter what the sport or activity. Others do whatever they can to avoid intense competition. They may be willing to challenge themselves, but they are unwilling to put themselves in a place where they might be evaluated and compared to others.

Most salespeople and athletes enjoy head-to-head competition; their problem is that they cannot shut off this tendency to be competitive. They have difficulty compromising; fail to realize that winning isn't everything; and forget that, under the right circumstances, they will accomplish more with cooperation than with competition.

Speed of Decision Making

Do you make decisions quickly, or do you prefer to deliberate first? Some individuals seem to make even the most complicated and important decisions quickly. Others seem to agonize over every little detail, apparently unable to take a firm stand on even the simplest of issues. Watch the way people play chess. One individual may begin a move before his or her opponent has finished; the other individual might take forever to make a move.

Differences in speed of decision making among individuals who work or live together can put a great deal of stress on relationships. The quick decision maker is stressed by not being able to move on; the slow decision maker is stressed by being pushed to move before he or she is ready. Such pressure affects concentration skills and emotional arousal and destroys performance and teamwork. Under pressure, quick decision makers will take risks and make errors of *commission* (deciding without all of the required data). Slow decision makers will delay and make errors of *omission*. The latter will often lose because they fail to take appropriate risks and to take advantage of unforeseen opportunities. These are the athletes who play not to lose, rather than playing to win.

Extroversion

Extroversion is the need for, and enjoyment of, involvement with other people. It is another performance-relevant and traitlike characteristic. Some performance situations require individuals to work in relative isolation; others require a great deal of socializing. Individuals who love to socialize sometimes struggle when they have to work alone. Under pressure, extroverts tend to seek out the involvement of others. If those others distract the extroverts rather than helping them to accomplish their objectives, extroversion can cause problems.

Introversion

Introversion is the need for, and enjoyment of, personal space and privacy. It can also be performance-relevant and traitlike. The more introverted an individual is, the more stressful that person will find situations that exclude personal space and privacy. Introverts are more comfortable in performance settings in which they can compete against themselves, typically in isolation. In sport, extreme introverts can have problems in team situations in which they face considerable pressure to be involved with other members of the team, both on and off the field. Under pressure, introverts tend to withdraw even more, thereby distancing themselves from people who might be able to help them.

Expressiveness

People differ dramatically in terms of their willingness to express thoughts and ideas, negative feelings and criticism, and positive feelings and support. Everyone encounters performance situations from time to time that require each of these types of expression. Some individuals are not expressive and score low in all three areas. Others are extremely comfortable expressing thoughts and ideas but are uncomfortable expressing feelings, positive or negative. Any combination of these three types of expression is possible. Many people are good at expressing positive feelings and support yet are seemingly unable to criticize others and to set limits. In sporting circles, we often come across coaches who are critical and confrontational but have little positive to say. We also meet coaches and athletes who are highly intellectual and verbal—future sportscasters, perhaps.

From interpersonal and intrapersonal standpoints, it is important to know something about a person's

- willingness to conform to the expectations of others,

- willingness and need to take responsibility and control,

- level of self-confidence and self-esteem,

- degree of interpersonal and personal competitiveness,

- speed of decision making,

- enjoyment of and need to be involved with others,

- desire and tolerance for personal space and privacy,

- willingness to express thoughts and ideas in front of others,

- willingness to confront and to set limits, and

- willingness to express to others thoughts and feelings of support and encouragement.

In addition to cognitive and interpersonal characteristics, we must have a sense of the individual's emotional state at the time of evaluation. A depressed person evaluates everything critically. Depression minimizes a person's strengths and maximizes weaknesses. When he or she is on an emotional high (e.g., after winning a championship), the reverse is true. This fact becomes important when we interpret test scores and try to place the resultant information in perspective.

Even when a problem seems to be narrow and our involvement will only be short-term, it helps to have the kind of information we've just discussed. For example, imagine trying to help a downhill skier get out of the starting gates faster. Before we begin to work with the individual, we would ask ourselves questions such as the following:

- Where is the room for improvement?

- Do we need to reduce the athlete's tendency to become externally distracted?

- Does the athlete have a low level of self-confidence, and is that contributing to negative thoughts and doubts (internal distractions)?

- If confidence and competitiveness are high, is the athlete tightening up physically because she is trying too hard, and is this what is slowing her down at the start?

- Is she too much of a critic, so high on negative expression and so low on positive expression that she can't see the positive and is continually frustrating herself?

- Does she see a need to improve?

- Is she willing and able to listen? (This will depend a great deal on her analytical skills, her need for control, and her level of self-confidence.)

- How much detail is she going to need and want in our communications with her?

- Should we keep our communications short and simple (low score in the analytical and intellectual expression areas), or will it help if we give her a more in-depth understanding of the reasons for our suggestions?

- Does she have the focus, self-discipline, and follow-through to practice and develop the psychological skills necessary for improvement without needing daily reminders from us?

- To what extent must we try to involve others in order to reduce distractions (e.g., to control her need to socialize) and keep her focused?

- Will she give up the control necessary to let someone (e.g., a coach or a teammate) help?

Of course, we could attain this information by spending significant time with the athlete and observing her behavior at competition, during practice, and in her daily interactions with others. This process, however, would be time consuming. With testing, we can get a preview of these areas in just a few minutes.

Predicting and controlling behavior are complex processes. You must know much more than someone's score on a single measure (e.g., anxiety, need to achieve, or degree of learned helplessness) to predict success or failure with any reasonable degree of accuracy. Individuals who are good at predicting behavior and at helping others have developed their own explicit or implicit sets of constructs that they use as guides. Whether you are consciously aware of it or not, you have already developed your own performance-relevant theory. You use it every day to make your own world a little more understandable and predictable. In this chapter, we have introduced you to the core constructs of our theory of performance.

The characteristics we have identified as performance-relevant should not be considered inherently good or bad; that would imply that individuals should have high or low scores. The usefulness of a behavior can be evaluated only within a performance context. What is good in one situation may be devastating in another.

Remember, too, that as pressure increases, an individual's dominant concentration and interpersonal skills become even more pronounced (Hull, 1952). The number of different performance demands the athlete can cope with effectively decreases as cognitive and interpersonal behaviors become less flexible. A thorough understanding of relative strengths (high scores) and weaknesses (low scores) in the areas we have discussed will help you to anticipate the mismatches between those characteristics and the demands of performance situations. This, in turn, will enable you to predict the circumstances that generate emotional arousal in an individual and to anticipate that individual's reaction to mismatches. Only then will you be capable of helping people to perform more effectively.

Examine the constructs you use to evaluate performance. Compare their effectiveness to the effectiveness of other explicit theoretical approaches. Consider letting go of some of your constructs and incorporating others into your existing theory. Be critical and look for exceptions to your theory; the behaviors not easily explained by your theory are often the ones most useful to explore.

To really challenge yourself, take time while you are reading and learning from this book to develop your own explicit and systematic theory of human performance. You can limit that theory to performance within a highly specific arena or apply it to performance across a broad spectrum. Don't stop, however, with the articulation of your theory; identify and develop some ways that you can more efficiently measure and evaluate the critical determinants of performance.

One of the difficulties in writing a book or teaching a course about the use of tests in sport is that limited time and space force a choice between presenting the available tools and teaching the assessment skills. Because the primary goal of this book is to help you develop assessment skills, we really cannot discuss the available assessment tools as much as we would like. However, the process you go through and the way you analyze, interpret, and evaluate information should be the same, independent of the test(s) you use to gather that information.

As you work through this book, do not limit yourself to our theory and instrument. Conduct your own review of the various tests used in sport. Evaluate those instruments as potential measures of the performance-relevant characteristics you believe to be important. Apply what you learn in this book to the assessment tools of your choice. In our classes, we ask students to search the Internet for psychological inventories that seem to measure the constructs they believe to be important predictors of performance. We then ask them to administer those instruments, as well as The Attentional and Interpersonal Style inventory, and to interpret and integrate information from all inventories into their reports.

Suggested Readings

Bacon, S. J. (1974). Arousal and the range of cue utilization. *Journal of Experimental Psychology, 103*, 81–87.

Csikszentmihalyi, M. (1990). *Flow: The psychology of optimal experience.* New York: Harper & Row.

Druckman, D., & Bjork, R. A. (Eds.). (1991). *In the mind's eye: Enhancing human performance.* Washington, DC: National Academy Press.

Easterbrook, J. A. (1959). The effect of emotion on cue utilization and the organization of behavior. *Psychological Review, 86*, 183–201.

Freud, S. (1940). An outline of psychoanalysis. *International Journal of Psychoanalysis, 21*, 27–84.

Garb, H. N. (1984). The incremental validity of information used in personality assessment. *Clinical Psychology Review, 4*, 641–655.

Heyman, S. R., & Anderson, M. B. (1998). When to refer athletes for counseling or psychotherapy. In J. M. Williams (Ed.), *Applied sport psychology* (pp. 359–371). Mountain View, CA: Mayfield.

Hull, C. L. (1952). *A behavior system.* New Haven: Yale University Press.

Landers, D. M., & Boutcher, S. H. (1998). Arousal-performance relationship. In J. M. Williams (Ed.), *Applied sport psychology* (pp. 197–218). Mountain View, CA: Mayfield.

Ludwig, A. (1969). Altered states of consciousness. In C. Tart (Ed.), *Altered states of consciousness.* New York: John Wiley & Sons.

Nideffer, R. M. (1976a). Altered states of consciousness. In T. X. Barber (Ed.), *Advanced in altered states of consciousness and human potentialities* (Vol. 1, pp. 3–36). New York: Psychological Dimensions.

Nideffer, R. M. (1976b). Test of attentional and interpersonal style. *Journal of Personality and Social Psychology, 34*, 394–404.

Nideffer, R. M. (1989). Theoretical and practical relationships between attention, anxiety, and performance in sport. In D. Hackfort & C. D. Spielberger (Eds.), *Anxiety in sport: An international perspective* (pp. 117–136). New York: Hemisphere Publishing.

Nideffer, R. M. (1992). *Psyched to win.* Champaign, IL: Leisure Press.

Nideffer, R. M. (1993). *Predicting human behavior: A theory and test of attentional and interpersonal style.* New Berlin, WI: Assessment Systems International.

Ostrow, A. (Ed.). (1996). *Directory of psychological tests in the sport and exercise sciences.* Morgantown, WV: Fitness Information Technology, Inc.

Selye, H. (1974). *Stress without distress.* New York: Lippincott.

Williams, J. M., & Krane V. (1998). Psychological characteristics of peak performance. In J. M. Williams (Ed.), *Applied sport psychology* (pp. 158–170). Mountain View, CA: Mayfield.

Yerkes, R. M., & Dodson, J. D. (1908). The relations of strength of stimulus to rapidity of habit formation. *Journal of Comparative Neurology of Psychology, 18*, 459–482.

The Importance of Consensual Validation

3

You can always pick the best kids out in our tryouts: They're the ones who jump right up after getting tackled and run back to the huddle.
—Pop Warner, football coach

A business executive once told us he based his hiring decisions on how quickly people moved from the reception area to his office. He believed the individuals who walked quickly were the ones who were motivated and driven. He didn't need any data other than that. Fortunately, we weren't looking for jobs; his approach might have made some sense to him, but it didn't make sense to us. (He must never have seen how slowly Jim Brown or Marcus Allen would get up and return to the huddle.)

It's easy to classify such comments as invalid and to see them as examples of personal bias. They do reflect a certain amount of bias, but any assessment process does. Validity is unavoidably based on the theoretical orientation of the assessor (bias, if you will). The assessor determines what will be observed and measured, and these decisions are a product of personal preferences.

This type of bias in measurement, however, does not make the measurement invalid (i.e., not predictive of behavior). Validity, as reported in journals and test manuals, is not an either/or event; it is a statistical, probabilistic concept. If the prediction of behavior by a test (or by a person's observation) is accurate more often than not, and if there are enough observations for statistical significance, the test is considered valid. This is true even if it is accurate as little as 51% of the time. Over the years, a coach may have observed a large number of players, and, on average, those who ran back to the huddle may indeed have been more motivated than those who did not run.

Even low predictive values can be extremely important under the right set of circumstances. If you know you are going to win the toss of a coin 51% of the time, you can make yourself rich. This is basically the case in Las Vegas, where they keep the slot machine player's odds for winning, and the corresponding cash payback, two or three percentage points below 50%. This way, the individual wins enough to keep playing but loses enough, over time, to make the casino rich.

When making decisions about a person's life, we would certainly like to be accurate more than 51% of the time; in fact, we would prefer 100% accuracy. However, given the complexity of human behavior and the influence of situational factors, it is impossible to be accurate 100% of the time, especially if we are relying on single measurements or observations of behavior.

Here is a sobering bit of information: The average validity coefficient for psychological inventories is somewhere between .3 and .4 (Mischel, 1968). This means that the inferences drawn from scores of subjects making up the validity study account for between 9% and 16% of the variance. It also means you increase your predictive accuracy above chance by 9% to 16%. If you were correct 50% of the time before using test data, you would now be accurate between 59% and 66% of the time. Prediction based on one set of data is far from perfect and necessitates the process of *consensual validation*.

Does this relatively low level of accuracy mean you shouldn't use psychological tests? We think not. Although we would like to be able to predict the outcome of individual events, expecting to do so is similar to expecting to win the lottery with only one ticket. There are too many things that can go wrong to allow us to have absolute faith in our ability to predict a single event.

You should not use a "blind" interpretation of a set of test scores as the sole criterion for making a decision. Any interpretation of test data based on a statistical formula (e.g., any computer-generated test report) is a blind interpretation. Any interpretation of test data made by a professional with no knowledge of the individual other than that provided by the test is also a blind interpretation.

We are not saying, "Don't make blind interpretations." We are saying, "Don't make decisions based solely on blind interpretations." The assessment process often begins with a blind interpretation. Many predictions begin with creative ideas or hunches. Making important decisions based on these types of unsupported predictions is dangerous; you will want to test, refine your ideas, and test again before you move too far ahead.

Those of us who use tests for assessment purposes make a living based on our ability to predict general tendencies or trends over time. Really, this is what interests us most. We are not as interested in predicting whether an athlete will be late to practice on Tuesday as we are in knowing whether that individual will be late to practice on a regular basis (Hogan, Hogan, & Roberts, 1996). A coach is more concerned about whether an individual has the characteristics necessary to win and to stay at the top over time than he or she is about the outcome of any individual competition. Luck may occasionally make someone a winner, but it never makes someone a champion. Because we are interested in predicting behavior over time, and in the development of consistency of performance, we don't rely solely on test information when making a decision. Instead, we use test information to highlight possible issues. We then collect additional information to enhance the likelihood that any inferences we draw, or any decisions we make, will be accurate.

Consensual Validation and the Generation of Behavioral Examples

When you use The Attentional and Interpersonal Style (TAIS) inventory, or any other psychological test, to make inferences about an individual, your effectiveness and accuracy depend on your ability to translate the constructs measured by the instrument into actual behaviors that are relevant to the athlete's performance. The ability to translate constructs into actual performance-relevant behaviors, to make them operational, is critical to the process of consensual validation and, ultimately, to the reliability and validity of your conclusions.

Let's look at the characteristics of *control* and *self-confidence* as measured by TAIS. Assume for the moment that an elite athlete and his coach both score extremely high on both factors. Based on our experience with the inventory, and on some of the validity and reliability studies that have been conducted, we might predict that as pressure increases, the athlete and the coach will experience a breakdown in their ability to communicate. We anticipate that under pressure, their confidence levels will affect their behavior by making them less willing to listen to opinions opposing their own. We predict that when disagreements occur, instead of hearing each other out, they will stop listening, become introspective, and begin trying to figure out how to convince one another that they are right. Because they are both confident and controlling, we predict that as pressure increases, so will their tendency to become angry and frustrated when they encounter disagreement; this will be apparent in their behavior. Communication will break down as they begin to argue, and they will have difficulty compromising.

Our behavioral inferences or hypotheses in this case are based on two sets of test scores. How accurate are these inferences? There is little doubt that if we wait long enough, our predictions will prove true. Any two people involved over a long period of time will become sensitive and stubborn at one point or another. What we need to know is just how frequently, and under what conditions, the behaviors we predict are likely to take place. To do this, we must find past examples of the behaviors. We will also want to observe the behaviors in process or create an interview situation that will elicit the predicted behaviors. We can do this only if we know what we're looking for and can anticipate how the behaviors will manifest themselves in various performance situations.

A few years ago, I was helping a graduate student develop his interviewing skills by having him participate in the selection of an undergraduate research assistant. I had advertised to find a student with a certain set of skills to work on an important project and had set up a series of interviews with applicants. The applicants were tested prior to the interview to help us determine whether they had the cognitive and interpersonal skills necessary to work effectively with the other members of the research team. I had taken the lead in interviewing several applicants, and the process was going smoothly.

On one particular interview, I suggested the graduate student take the lead. I told him the test scores suggested that the individual he was to interview might be a little too controlling and verbal for the group; it would be important for us to explore this in the interview. The student left the interview room to introduce himself to the applicant, then brought him back into the room. The seating arrangement was contructed to communicate a clear hierarchy. I had moved to the side and left the "interviewer's" chair vacant for the graduate student. As the two entered the room, the applicant immediately strode across the room, introduced himself to me, and asked, "Who are you?" He then took the interviewer's seat and proceeded to pull out a tape recorder, saying, "You don't mind if I tape this, do you?" Without waiting for a response, he turned his tape recorder on and began to interview us. The graduate student was so shocked he just sat there and allowed the applicant to take complete control of the interview process.

The applicant, without any prompting, had consensually validated our concerns. His behavior in the interview was exactly what we would have predicted on the basis of test scores. As a result, he gave us the information we needed to make our decision (we rejected him). Other applicants had scored as high as this individual on self-esteem and the need for control but had exhibited considerably more control over their behavior; consequently, they were more likely to be successful in the position we were seeking to fill.

If you really want to improve your ability to understand, predict, and control behavior, then follow these tips:

- Choose tests that measure performance-relevant constructs, constructs that are easy to translate into observable behaviors.

- Choose tests that measure several different performance-relevant constructs, or choose several tests that measure different individual constructs. One construct (e.g., anxiety) can't explain performance across different individuals and different situations. You must measure enough distinct cognitive and interpersonal characteristics to begin to take into account the influences that individual and situational differences have on performance. For example, some highly anxious people perform very well under pressure. You will want to find out why. To do that, you need to discover the *mediating* variables; that is, the variables that interact with the individuals' high level of anxiety, allowing him or her to perform well in spite of that anxiety. You can't discover these variables if you only measure anxiety.

- Translate each construct measured into behavior you would expect to see in an interview with the person. This is critical to the process of consensual validation and will help you to define the conditions under which a predicted behavior is more or less likely to manifest itself.

- Translate each construct measured into behaviors you would expect to see if you were observing the individual perform in his or her particular performance arena. For instance, how might a midfielder in soccer behave when highly anxious? How would you expect a controlling gymnastics coach to act at a major competition?

- Create conditions that allow you to observe the individual's behavior under varying degrees of pressure and arousal. Remember: Most people can remain fairly flexible and can control even their dominant behaviors when they aren't under serious pressure. You want to see how much difference increasing pressure makes.

Table 3 lists the various constructs measured by TAIS. Take the time to translate these constructs into actual behaviors, both in the interview and in a specific performance situation. Discuss your examples with others and engage in this same process with any other instrument you may be using or developing.

Table 3. Behavioral Descriptions of TAIS Constructs

TAIS scale	*Behavioral examples of the construct expected in an interview.*	*Behavioral examples of the construct expected when performing.*
BET: Externally aware. Sensitive to the moods and feelings of others. Good "street sense."		
OET: External distractibility. Sensitivity to task-*irrelevant* environmental cues.		
BIT: Analytical/conceptual ability. Ability to analyze and plan.		
OIT: Internal distractibility. Tendency to become overloaded by thoughts and feelings.		
NAR: Ability to focus attention and willingness to pay attention to details.		
RED: Tendency to (a) become lost in thoughts, (b) lose awareness of the environment, and (c) react to the environment without adequate thought.		
INFP: Information-processing capacity. Ability to multitask. Need for change. Enjoyment of a busy environment.		
BCON: Willingness to deviate from the norm or "do one's own thing." May also indicate behavioral impulsivity and loss of control over anger.		
CON: Need for control. Desire and willingness to assume responsibility for self and others.		
SES: Self-confidence. Belief in one's abilities. Self-esteem. Belief in one's value as a person.		

Table 3. Behavioral Descriptions of TAIS Constructs (Continued)

TAIS scale	Behavioral examples of the construct expected in an interview.	Behavioral examples of the construct expected when performing.
P/O: Physical orientation. Enjoyment of physical competition and willingness to engage in head-to-head competition.		
OBS: Provides an indication of the speed with which an individual makes decisions.		
EXT: Extroversion. The enjoyment of, and need for, involvement with others.		
INT: Introversion. The enjoyment of, and need for, time alone, personal space, and privacy.		
IEX: Intellectual expressiveness. The willingness and need to express thoughts and ideas in front of others.		
NAE: Negative affect expression. The willingness to confront and challenge the thoughts and actions of others.		
PAE: Positive affect expression. The willingness and ability to express support and encouragement to others.		
DEP: Depression/self-criticalness. Indicates the individual's mood at the time of testing.		

Ethical and Professional Considerations

The process of consensual validation, of verifying the inferences you are making based on test information (e.g., through interview or through observable behaviors), is a professional responsibility you must take seriously. Because this process raises some important issues, the following questions might be helpful to consider:

- Should your attempts at using information from one place (e.g., tests) to consensually validate behaviors seen in another place (e.g., an interview) be completely independent of each other? Or should you use what you learn about an individual through a test to help determine what you should look for in the interview, and vice versa?

- When information from one source is inconsistent with, and therefore does not consensually validate, information from another source, how do you know what, if any, information to trust?

- Should you have information from a person's test responses when you interview him or her?

- Are you afraid that knowing, or thinking you know, something about a person's behavior in advance will cause you to see the behavior even if it isn't there?

- Are you afraid that test information will prejudice you?

We've known athletes who have been labeled as chokers on the basis of a single poor performance. Many of them were never given a second chance to prove the label wrong. With these scarlet-letter athletes, even minor mistakes become evidence of the label. Tragically, some of these athletes applied the "choking" label to their own behavior. Consider the following examples:

- Suppose you are working with a team and the coach asks you for help with an athlete. The coach tells you that communication with the athlete has broken down. He says that the athlete has a great deal of talent but is stubborn and will not listen, and he wants you to talk with her to find out what the problem is. What are you going to do? Have you already been biased by the information provided by the coach?

- Jim has been suspended for six games right at the end of the season because of repeated rules violations. All of the violations occurred during games, and all of them were a direct result of Jim losing control over his emotions. Jim has come to you on his own for help. He loves the game, he cares about the team, and he realizes that his anger is getting in the way. Are you biased as you enter your first session with Jim?

- A coach has told you that her team needs some help with the "mental side of the game," and she has given you a 1½-hour block of time between lectures on nutrition and stretching to make a presentation. Are you entering that situation biased?

- You are acting as a mental talent scout for a National Football League team that is participating in the draft. You have been asked to help them identify the players who are mentally tough and those who are not. Are you biased?

If you answered yes to any of these questions, don't be surprised; bias is unavoidable. There is always information available to you when you formulate judgments and make decisions. This information limits your choices and the elements you consider. The question is, how can you be sure that those limitations don't interfere with responsible, ethical decision making? You can't do it by refusing exposure to past, performance-relevant information.

To make responsible decisions, you must first be aware of relevant background information and the current performance context; then, you must attach an appropriate weight to that information. How reliable is it? Have you evaluated it critically? Have you kept an open mind with respect to new information? Judgment is always a matter of examining old evidence in the face of new evidence and vice versa. Prejudice occurs when you either fail to examine old evidence in a critical way or close your mind to new evidence. Prejudice is undesirable, unexamined bias.

We believe that information from testing should be available and that you should employ it in structuring the interview process. This is the most effective way to consensually validate the inferences you draw from test information. Testing should precede the interview, rather than the other way around, because you then have greater flexibility in the interview process. It is easier to adjust the interview to the test results than it is to do the reverse.

Bias

Bias is present, to a greater or lesser degree, in every decision people make. Performance-relevant characteristics and behaviors should be considered good or bad only within a situational context. Your role as a professional is to help place behaviors into appropriate situational contexts. Under what conditions do certain behaviors appear? When they appear, are they appropriate for the situation? If they are appropriate, then they are desirable. If they are not appropriate, then they are undesirable. The issue is practical, not emotional.

Putting behaviors into a situational context is not only critical for controlling bias but also should form the basis for any intervention or training program you develop. Unless the expression of a behavior that you are trying to help an individual control is predictable, you won't have much hope of influencing it, nor will you have any assurance that the behavior is anything but a random act.

Do not allow yourself to draw conclusions in the absence of actual data. Behaviors that may be very highly correlated with the behaviors of an entire group, team, or class of individuals may not apply to everyone in that group, team, or class. Typically, test scores lead to inferences about behavior. We might see one score indicating an individual becomes distracted by thoughts and feelings, another score indicating a lack of self-confidence, and a third score suggesting the person is slow to make decisions. On the basis of these three scores, we infer that when time is running out in a close competition, this person will freeze.

We have just made a series of logical inferences about behavior not yet actually observed. Research testing the validity of these inferences might have demonstrated their statistical validity; remember, however, that the validity coefficient obtained in any study, no matter how significant, will be nowhere near perfect. Even within the original validation group, it was probably accurate only about 65% of the time. Furthermore, there will be important differences between the actual testing situation and the one in which the validity of your inference was evaluated. There may also be important educational, biological, genetic, ethnic, and cultural differences between your subject and the other individuals. All of these factors affect your ability to generalize. Before you draw any conclusions, observe the behavior and identify a predictable pattern or specific set of circumstances that seems to elicit the behavior.

Test yourself first. If you have not taken TAIS, now is the time to do so. If you have other instruments you are using and you have not taken those, now is the time. The best way to protect the people you serve is to increase your own self-awareness. How do your attitudes and behaviors differ from those of the people around you? When are you more likely to jump to inappropriate conclusions? When do your emotions prevent you from keeping the things you see in the proper perspective? Until you have insight into your own tendencies and abilities, you won't be able to discount your own prejudices effectively. All people see the world through unique lenses. It is important to know how these lenses shape what is seen. "Know thyself" is not just some ancient Greek maxim; it is a powerful call to learn about how you view the world.

Challenge your own conclusions before you allow yourself or anyone else to act upon them. When you have more than one option or interpretation available to you, question your motives for making the choice that you make. Whose interests are you considering? Would others see you as responding to your own needs, or to those of your client?

Dealing With Inconsistent Data

What happens when the information you get from a test doesn't fit with what you know about the person or with the reports other people have given you? Does it mean that one set of data is right and the other is wrong? Could both be wrong? Sometimes a piece of information is inaccurate. More often than not, however, it isn't so simple; the complexity of the assessment process is what makes it so challenging.

Your mother probably sees you as a charming, lovable person who can do no wrong. Your worst critic probably sees you as totally incompetent. Where is the truth? On whose opinions should you rely, and under what circumstances?

Remember John in chapter 1? At first blush, his test information seemed inconsistent with the observations and experiences of his coach. John's stellar sprinting performances and seemingly positive interactions with his coach gave no outward indication that anything was wrong. John's test information, however, taken in the absence of any knowledge about John's actual ability to perform, seemed to indicate that nothing was right. Both pieces of information were valid descriptions of John: One described his performance on the track, and the other described his feelings about himself and his situation.

Sport-Specific Versus More General Measures of Performance

The apparent inconsistency between John's test scores and his coach's observations brings up an interesting issue. Should the assessment tools you use be sport-specific? Should the items focus on the actual behavior within the situational context that interests you? If this had been the case with John and the questions on his tests, the coach might never have discovered how unhappy John was. A highly structured, situation-specific inventory might have led John to describe his behavior as others saw it or in such a narrow way as to miss larger issues. At the time John was assessed, would specific information about John's performance have helped the coach? We doubt it. The coach had had 2 full years with John. He knew how well John could perform, and he did not need a psychological test to help predict John's behavior on the track. What the coach needed was a better understanding of John—a way to find out what made him tick. What could be done to make him an even better, more consistent performer? The coach needed to understand John as a person, not just as a 100-meter sprinter.

Although we have emphasized the importance of being practical rather than emotional when making decisions based on situational factors, we don't mean to suggest that legal, moral, and ethical factors don't play a role. As a professional, you will sometimes have serious questions about whether you want to provide the kind of information a coach or an athlete is requesting. Typically, your discomfort will be based on your ethical beliefs and moral values, rather than on practical issues. Professional guidelines will often leave these decisions to you, but you must be prepared to justify your course of action. For practice, consider the following situation:

> You have been asked to provide psychological information that will be part of the data a team is using to make decisions during the draft. You have tested, interviewed, and reviewed the histories of two equally gifted athletes. The only difference you can see between the two athletes is their test scores. One athlete's scores indicate he is more likely than the other to perform poorly under pressure. You have attempted to find evidence supporting this difference in the interview and through a careful examination of the athlete's history, but have been unable to do so. What information will you provide to the decision makers?

Suggested Readings

Eyde, L. D., Robertson, G. J., Krug, S. E., Moreland, K. L., Robertson, A. G., Shewan, C. M., Harrison, P. L., Porch, B. E., Hammer, A. L., & Primoff, E. S. (1993). *Responsible test use: Case studies for assessing human behavior.* Washington, DC: American Psychological Association.

Hogan, R., Hogan, J., & Roberts, B. W. (1996). Personality measurement and employment decisions, questions and answers. *American Psychologist, 51,* 469–477.

Mischel, W. (1968). *Personality and assessment.* New York: Wiley.

American Psychological Association. (1985). *Standards for educational and psychological testing.* Washington, DC: Author.

Operationalizing the Referral 4

When coaches or athletes resist talking to a sport psychologist, their resistance usually reflects their fear that the psychologist will create more problems than he or she solves. It isn't that coaches and athletes feel mental factors are unimportant; many of them think mental factors are more important than we do. They worry because they know how susceptible most athletes are to overthinking and to becoming distracted by negative thoughts, doubts, and fears. They also know that psychologists have a tendency to approach things from a clinical perspective and to inquire into highly personal material. They worry that this approach, aside from causing discomfort, will do more harm than good. Some coaches and athletes believe mental training and assessment are a waste of time. To them, a person either is mentally tough or is not. Because there is usually more than enough technical and tactical training to be done, taking time away from important issues would be stupid, in their opinion.

To deal successfully with these legitimate concerns of many coaches and athletes, you must

- provide a convincing reason for testing and assessment,

- clearly define why you have chosen to use certain instruments, and

- explain how test information will be used to accomplish client goals and objectives.

Testing, under most circumstances, should not be a fishing expedition. Whenever you engage in testing, you should have a reason. Your reason should serve to structure and guide the assessment process. We call the process of establishing an initial structure *operationalizing the reason for referral*. It is really just behaviorally defining the goals and objectives behind the testing. This process should begin when you first meet with your client. Behaviorally defining your goals and demonstrating the link between those goals and the process you are asking the client to go through are critical to gaining the client's respect, trust, and cooperation.

Program Adherence

From this chapter on, the material in the book will be presented in an increasingly systematic and sequential way. As you move from chapter to chapter, we will ask you to analyze, to solve problems, and to make predictions. Some of you will be tempted to read ahead, either to find out the answers or to check your own thought processes before investing time in the exercise. Please don't do that. We have tried to organize this book in a way that will help you develop your assessment skills. If you read ahead, no matter what your motive, you defeat one of the main purposes of the book. Because this point is so important to us, we have decided to make our case below for NOT peeking:

- Reading ahead to find our answers is like cheating on an exam in class. If you haven't studied, how do you know if the other person's answer is correct? Even if our answers are good ones, they may not be the best or the only good answers. You may think of a better answer, and we don't want you to give up too easily.

- Reading ahead denies you the opportunity to make mistakes. Like the athletes we all work with, we learn from making mistakes, not from error-free performance. Practice what you preach.

- Reading ahead limits your opportunity to develop and defend your own thought processes. The concepts and problems you have worked through yourself are the ones you are most likely to remember and to benefit from in the future.

- Reading ahead limits your opportunity to predict our behavior. How far into this book are you going to have to read before you are able to assess us, anticipating and predicting our thought processes and the positions we take on issues?

Choosing Your Clients

When people approach us for help, whether over the telephone, in person, or through a friend or acquaintance, we first want to determine whether they have approached the right person/company. We have found that many people who contact us believe that sport psychology is the answer to all their problems. It's not that they have too little faith in sport psychology, but that they have too much.

Some people contact us when they have reached normal developmental plateaus. To get to the next level, these individuals need time and practice, not a sport psychologist. Still others contact us because they think they should. They have read an article about sport psychology and found it intriguing. Coaches come to us because they can't seem to get their athletes to listen or to follow instructions; they think that we can get those athletes to comply. Athletes who need clinical help approach us, but this is not our area of specialization. Finally, people contact us with issues of which we have no understanding or in which we have little interest.

Helping others to improve performance and to communicate more effectively is not brain surgery. You don't usually have to be the world's greatest expert in an area to help. You must, however, have a genuine interest in the individual and an ability to win that person's trust and confidence. Don't fake it. If you can't relate to the person, can't define a role that makes sense, don't have an interest, or don't respect the person's goals and objectives, don't get involved.

You will find that most of the people who come to you for help have difficulty defining what they think you can provide. They need your help in clarifying and defining the issues. Throughout this chapter, we will provide examples of the kinds of requests we receive. Read them, and then do the following for each one:

1. Write down your first impressions or the first serious question that comes to mind regarding the referral.

2. Write down what led to your first thought or question.

3. Indicate how your reaction to the referral is apt to dictate your next steps, how it influences your perception of the problem, and how it is likely to affect your treatment of the athlete.

Referral 1

You receive a call from Sam, a Major League second baseman. He tells you he is playing in the World Series and asks if you saw last night's game. When you tell him you did not, he says that if you had, you would know why he's calling: "We lost the third game last night because of an error I made in the ninth inning. I choked big time, and I need your help."

What are your first thoughts?

_____

_____

_____

_____

What previous experiences and what information given in the brief reason for referral led to your above response?

_____

_____

_____

_____

How would your thoughts and feelings direct your involvement in any future assessment work?

_____

_____

_____

_____

Referral 2

The head of player development for a professional team calls and asks you to do a psychological evaluation on an athlete the team is considering acquiring in a trade. This is the first contact you have ever had with this particular organization.

What are your first thoughts?

_____

_____

_____

_____

What previous experiences and what information given in the brief reason for referral led to your above response?

_____

_____

_____

_____

How would your thoughts and feelings direct your involvement in any future assessment work?

_____

_____

_____

_____

Referral 3

Marge, the mother of a nationally ranked, 15-year-old tennis player named Tina, calls for an appointment. She tells you that her daughter's high school coach read a book on sport psychology. She has been talking with the coach about her daughter's progress, and the coach believes it might be helpful for Tina to talk with a sport psychologist.

What are your first thoughts?

_____

_____

_____

_____

What previous experiences and what information given in the brief reason for referral led to your above response?

_____

_____

_____

_____

How would your thoughts and feelings direct your involvement in any future assessment work?

_____

_____

_____

_____

Referral 4

It is 4 months before the Olympic trials. You are observing a regional diving competition when Debbie, a 24-year-old, world-class, 10-meter tower diver asks if she can talk to you. She says she knows you are a sport psychologist and she thinks you might be able to help her overcome her fear of a reverse 2½ somersault.

What are your first thoughts?

_____

_____

_____

_____

What previous experiences and what information given in the brief reason for referral led to your above response?

_____

_____

_____

_____

How would your thoughts and feelings direct your involvement in any future assessment work?

_____

_____

_____

_____

Referral 5

You receive a call from Pete, a 42 year old who describes himself as a "rapid-fire pistol shooter with 3 years of competitive experience." He tells you that his goal is to make the national team. He asks if you have any previous experience with shooters and then, without waiting for you to answer, informs you that "shooting is as much a mental game as it is a physical one." Pete goes on to say that he is a very thorough person and wants an appointment to talk to you just to make sure he's covered everything.

What are your first thoughts?

_____

_____

_____

_____

What previous experiences and what information given in the brief reason for referral led to your above response?

_____

_____

_____

_____

How would your thoughts and feelings direct your involvement in any future assessment work?

_____

_____

_____

_____

Referral 6

Natasha, a 30-year-old professional athlete, comes to you complaining about concentration problems and moodiness. She tells you that most of the time she has relatively few problems and a great relationship with her teammates and coach but that every once in a while, she gets a little crazy and hard to deal with.

What are your first thoughts?

_____

_____

_____

_____

What previous experiences and what information given in the brief reason for referral led to your above response?

_____

_____

_____

_____

How would your thoughts and feelings direct your involvement in any future assessment work?

_____

_____

_____

_____

Referral 7

Oscar, an Olympic coach, calls and says he would like you to test all of the athletes he's working with. He and his teams have been tested in the past and have found the resultant information to be very helpful. The athletes have about 6 weeks to prepare for the Olympic trials, and Oscar wants them to perform as well as they can.

What are your first thoughts?

_____

_____

_____

_____

What previous experiences and what information given in the brief reason for referral led to your above response?

_____

_____

_____

_____

How would your thoughts and feelings direct your involvement in any future assessment work?

_____

_____

_____

_____

Referral 8

The parent of a 10-year-old asks you to work with his son, Bobby. Bobby is having problems in school. Despite recommendations of counseling, Bobby refuses to see a psychologist. Because Bobby is a sports fan and a reasonable athlete, his father thinks he will consent to see you.

What are your first thoughts?

_____

_____

_____

_____

What previous experiences and what information given in the brief reason for referral led to your above response?

_____

_____

_____

_____

How would your thoughts and feelings direct your involvement in any future assessment work?

_____

_____

_____

_____

Referral 9

You receive a call from a basketball coach asking you to evaluate Dirk, a 20-year-old athlete who has a tremendous amount of talent but hasn't lived up to his potential. The athlete is currently recovering from an automobile accident and is undergoing mandatory counseling for driving while under the influence of alcohol.

What are your first thoughts?

_____

_____

_____

_____

What previous experiences and what information given in the brief reason for referral led to your above response?

_____

_____

_____

_____

How would your thoughts and feelings direct your involvement in any future assessment work?

_____

_____

_____

_____

Referral 1—An Error at Second Base

First Impressions

My first impression of Sam was that he was overreacting to something that could have happened to anyone. This made me wonder how he got my name.

Impressions

Making an error at second base, even if the error occurs in a big game, doesn't make an athlete a choker. Unless there is a pattern to the mistake, and unless the mistake leads to a downward performance spiral (e.g., additional errors in the game), it isn't choking. It is highly unlikely the team would be in the World Series at all if this athlete were playing second base and were a choker.

I knew through experience that it is not unusual for highly competitive athletes to become emotionally upset and take more than their share of the blame for a loss. Usually, however, these emotions are expressed as frustration, rage, and anger. When this is the response, the athlete beats himself up verbally and swears it will never happen again. Most athletes are too proud and too confident to ask for help. Unusual in this case were the request for help and the emotional response of anxiety rather than anger.

That Sam was seeking help indicated he was afraid he would make the same mistake again. Experience suggested that in this instance, a request for help was a bad sign. It takes a great deal of anxiety to drive a professional baseball player to seek out a sport psychologist in the middle of a World Series—enough anxiety to significantly enhance the likelihood of further difficulties concentrating and executing at second base.

The tight timelines (his next game was that afternoon) and high level of anxiety made this a crisis situation. His request made it clear he had lost confidence in himself. I was supposed to be the magician who would restore his confidence. In order for that to happen, he would have to already have, or to quickly develop, a great deal of faith and confidence in me and in my ability to help him. Knowing how he came to contact me would help me to determine the level of his confidence in my ability.

Implications

Because Sam was in the middle of the World Series, the last thing he needed was for me to feed his fear of being a choker or to probe for problems. Testing under such conditions would make no sense at all. There was no time for testing, and adding information to a system already overloaded due to anxiety would only confuse things and make matters worse.

In 1–2 hours, I needed to (a) calm Sam down enough to get him to express his fear as directly as he could, and still keep the discussion focused on the upcoming game; (b) encourage him to be completely candid so he would know that any direction I provided was given with full knowledge of the problem; (c) build his confidence in me and in what I would tell him; (d) convince him that he wasn't a choker; and (e) persuade him that his skills were still intact. Also, I needed to give him something he could focus on during the game that would help him to regain an appropriate mode of concentration and emotional control.

Answers to the Questions, and Resolution

Sam had heard me make a presentation on concentration when he was with another team. At that time, the coach had introduced me as "knowing more about concentration and performance than anyone in the world." The coach emphasized to his players that he would not get anyone who "wasn't the best" involved with the team. I could not have asked for a more supportive introduction.

I managed to find a 90-minute block of time when I could meet with Sam before he had to rejoin the team. Prior to our meeting, I read the newspapers to find out how the error had been reported in the press. As I suspected, the press believed it had contributed to the outcome of the game, but no one was labeling Sam a choker.

I spent the first 15 minutes listening to Sam describe his thoughts and feelings just before the error, during the play, and then for the remainder of the game. Throughout, I listened to him and empathized with how badly he felt, considering the significance of his error. In essence, I helped him to see that his feelings about the error were normal: "I've dealt with hundreds of athletes in these kinds of situations, and they all have had similar feelings. That's an indication of how much you care about the game and your team. I wouldn't want to be working with someone who cared any less than you obviously do."

His anxiety indicated he was afraid his feelings would lead to more mistakes. Although that was possible, I was not going to tell him that. If he could accept his feelings as normal, he could let them go, and they wouldn't interfere with subsequent performance.

In describing his error, he told me that he had rushed. Because of the importance of the situation and the fact that the runner on first was one of the faster players in the league, he had looked up just a fraction of a second early. He misjudged the hop of the ball, which bounced off the end of his glove and dribbled out into center field. Instead of an inning-ending double play, one run scored, and the runner at first made it to third. The runner on third scored before the inning was over. Sam's team failed to score in the bottom of the ninth, and that was it.

I helped him to understand how his thoughts affected his physical responses, so he could see exactly how the error had occurred. I emphasized that the link between thoughts and physiology is normal; and I reminded him that he had made similar errors before, for the same reasons, and that he had always recovered from them.

I was very confident about the things I was saying to him, and I expressed a great deal of confidence in him. I told him that if he did find himself worrying during the game, he could control it by focusing on the ball and "talking it into his glove." His team ultimately lost the series, but he played well during the remaining games. I never heard from him again.

Referral 2—An Athlete in a Trade

First Impressions

First, we wanted to know whether getting a psychological evaluation on a player was standard operating procedure for this team.

Reasons for Our Question, and Implications

Because this was a first contact, we needed to know the team's expectations. If a psychological evaluation was a routine part of the team's selection process, the expectations would be fairly firm and would include information such as the type(s) of assessment devices we would employ and the general structure and format of any report we would provide.

If the organization had been using some other group to provide assessment services prior to this, we wanted to know why the team was switching. This information would be critical in deciding whether we would take the assignment and, if we did take it, in avoiding the types of problems that had led the team to switch to a new service provider. If the team had never used a psychological evaluation before, why had the team felt it necessary in this particular case? Experience suggests that most sports organizations do not make changes or try new approaches easily; this is especially true within the psychological arena. The odds are high that if a psychological evaluation is being considered for the first time, the person you will test has, or has had, a serious problem. The most likely problem would be one of alcohol or drug abuse. The second most likely problem would be anxiety associated with injuries and injury recovery.

Answer to Our Question

Psychological assessment was not a routine procedure for this team. When we asked why they wanted testing for this particular athlete, the team said it was because he had been caught using drugs. He had been in rehab programs on two different occasions. The latest drug tests indicated he was "clean," but the team officials were still concerned.

The player was one of the most physically gifted athletes in the league—so gifted, in fact, that he could turn an entire team around. Problems had occurred in the past because he had become involved with the wrong people and because he seemed to feel his talents meant that he did not have to play by the same rules as everyone else did. He missed practices every once in a while and frequently failed to work as hard as the coaches would have liked.

The owners and coaches of the new team hoped that a different environment and some positive support would be enough to keep this athlete out of trouble. They contacted us because they knew we had helped another team make some personnel decisions. They heard that testing had been helpful in that process, but they knew nothing about the testing or about the tests that were used. They believed that test information would tell them whether they were making the right decision about this trade.

Referral 3—A 15-Year-Old Tennis Player

First Impressions

I was curious: Was there an identified problem? Did Tina want to talk to a sport psychologist?

Reasons for My Questions

Over the past 20 years, many individuals have come to me because they have come across one of my books. Fewer than 5% of these calls are simply about wanting to learn more about what I do. The majority of the time, people pick up a book because there is an issue, and they call because the book has apparently offered some hope.

Another interesting thing I have learned over the years is that the person who reads a self-help book (at least, the first person) is not always the one with the problem. The person who reads the book first is often someone who is concerned about the individual with the problem. I have also learned that the individual concerned about the person with the problem is usually a big part of that problem.

Implications

If there were no problems, I had to decide whether getting involved with Tina made sense. Would an appointment with me be a good use of her time? If there weren't any problems, and her progress would not be impaired by studying sport psychology, then it was up to me to decide whether I wanted to spend my time teaching her about it. If there was a problem, It was important that I identify it and determine the extent to which Tina, her coach, and Marge agreed on its nature and severity. If a problem did exist, I could be of help to Tina only if she perceived a problem and if she saw me as her ally, not as an agent of her mother or of the coach.

Answers to My Questions

Marge indicated that as far as she was concerned there was no problem. She didn't believe the coach saw a problem either. She didn't really know how sport psychology would help, and she had made contact with me because the coach thought it might be helpful and because her daughter seemed eager to talk to me. She said she was just doing what any mother would do—trying to help. Marge was surprised by my questions and seemed confused. She had taken it on faith that seeing a sport psychologist was a good idea, but now she wasn't sure. She suggested I call the coach and talk to him.

When I called the coach, he said he had worked with several players who had been successful on the professional circuit. This young woman was "the best of them all." She had a 4.0 grade point average and was intent on going to Stanford University. She was a great person in every way. No one had a more positive attitude or worked any harder. She could be and do anything she wanted. The coach believed Tina would graduate from college and still rank among the top 10 in the world. She was "psychologically minded," and as far as the coach was concerned, now was the time for her to develop the psychological skills that could help her maximize her talent.

Referral 4—Fear of a Reverse 2½

First Impressions

The following questions came to mind when we considered this referral: How did the fear Debbie associated with this dive differ from the fear she had experienced with other dives? Was her coach supportive of her talking to us?

Reasons for Our Questions

Diving is a high-risk sport, and fear is an everyday experience for most elite-level divers. A 24-year-old competing at a national level has had to overcome fear along the way. The immediate competitive situation was not one that we would have expected to generate significant anxiety. Debbie was world-class and, for her, this was a low level of competition.

Because diving is such a high-risk sport, there is usually a very close relationship between diver and coach. Most elite-level coaches don't like giving up any control (e.g., to a psychologist). They feel that the best way to treat fear on the tower is to face it directly, not to run away from it.

Implications

Fear is a response to a perceived threat, and part of that response is a tensing of muscles, which can interfere dramatically with a diver's fine-motor coordination and timing. In high-risk sports like diving and gymnastics, unchecked fear can become a self-fulfilling prophecy. Changes in muscle tension due to anxiety and fear lead to the very mistakes the person is afraid of making.

It was essential that we find out whether the fear Debbie was experiencing differed from the fear she had with other dives. This would help us to determine whether her fear was normal. If it was similar to the fear she felt with other dives, she would probably only need some reassurance; however, if the fear was unlike what she experienced with other dives, this problem would require some clinical skills and background. If this wasn't typical fear, then using willpower to face it and to overcome it probably wouldn't be a good approach. If the coach wasn't supportive of Debbie talking to us or if he couldn't support any of our recommendations, we wouldn't be able to do much.

Answers to Our Questions

According to Debbie, the coach supported her consultation with us. He was supportive because he felt the fear was "stupid" and thought that somehow we could make Debbie see that. As we talked, Debbie indicated that her fear was different in this case because it wasn't going away. She was afraid of hitting her head on the tower: "I just know I'm going to hit the tower. I can see myself hitting it. I'm afraid I'm going to kill myself on this dive."

She had successfully executed a reverse 2½ somersault during competition for several months. Her problems occurred during practice. At those times, her fear kept her from performing the dive, and this was creating major problems with her coach. He would yell and scream; she would stall and cry. During a competition, she knew she had to do the dive and would somehow force herself to do it.

When we asked if she had encountered similar experiences in the past, Debbie mentioned that she had been an extremely gifted musician as a young child. As her musical talent developed, however, the pressure to perform well also increased. At the age of 10, she experienced a breakdown and had not played since. She was afraid the same thing would happen with diving.

Referral 5—Rapid-Fire Pistol Shooting

First Impressions

We had some initial questions: What made Pete think he could compete at a national level? Would he listen to us and follow any suggestions we might make?

Reasons for Our Questions

In contrast to many of our referrals, Pete had a very specific goal or objective in mind: He wanted to make the national team. Not knowing much about rapid-fire pistol shooting, we first had to determine how realistic his goal was; then, we had to learn more about the physical and psychological requirements for success on a national level in his sport.

Pete said he had only been shooting competitively for 3 years. Talented individuals can achieve fairly high levels of performance rapidly in closed-skill sports like archery, shooting, and golf. There is a great deal of room for improvement early on, and because of this, many athletes think they have the talent to excel. The difference between good golfers and great golfers, or good shooters and great shooters, may be small in terms of points or number of strokes per round, but it is huge in terms of consistency of performance over time.

Our second question grew out of our awareness that Pete was extremely controlling and almost arrogant in the way he presented himself and the issues. He knew what he wanted to accomplish. He didn't ask us if psychology was important; he told us it was. He did ask a question about our respective backgrounds and experience, but he didn't give us time to answer. It was as if our answers were irrelevant. He knew what he needed, and he would decide whether or not we had anything to offer. Finally, he asked for an appointment. He didn't ask if an appointment would be appropriate; to him, that was not a point for discussion. He wanted an appointment, and he felt it was our responsibility to comply.

Implications

If our assumption about Pete's need to be in control was correct, we would have to do more listening than talking. We would have to work hard to earn his respect and to get him to listen, especially when his opinions differed from ours. We had to be mindful of our own limitations and lack of knowledge. Even if we were sure we knew something that he did not know about improving his shooting, it was important that we remember to qualify our opinions and ideas by deferring to his higher level of expertise. For example, *"We know what we're saying applies to diving, and it fits with our understanding of your situation, but you're the shooting expert. What do you think?"* To be effective with highly controlling individuals, you must convey confidence in what you know and equal confidence in what you do not know. This would be a challenge with Pete. With a person like him, you can't afford to be seen as defensive, and you can't afford to become involved in power struggles.

Answers to Our Questions

When we asked Pete how realistic his goal was, he gave us a very long and detailed answer. It was obvious from his presentation that he had thought a great deal about the issue, and he wanted us to know that. He began by giving us background information and history. He told us that he had been an excellent athlete in college, competing at a very high level in both soccer and rowing. His one regret as an intercollegiate athlete was that he had never made a national team. He enlisted in the Marines right after college, and during that period he realized he had some talent as a shooter, though he didn't do any competitive shooting.

After leaving the service, he married and began selling computer software. He made a reasonable living but was not happy; he still had a burning desire to make a national team. He decided to set a goal to accomplish this: He would organize the rest of his life around making a national squad. He selected rapid-fire pistol shooting because he had demonstrated some talent in this during his military service and his age, though a factor, would be of minor importance. Furthermore, the United States had a relatively weak team. Though he might not have ranked as competitive in some other countries, the U.S. program was poorly developed, and he believed he had a chance here.

Because the U.S. program was not well funded and because he was older, he knew he would have to support himself. That meant he would have to build a training facility and to hire his own coach. Supporting his shooting would require a lot of money. He carefully analyzed his skills and the business environment and decided the best way to make the kind of money he needed was as a software publisher.

Pete developed a business plan and a budget. He and his wife took out a $10,000 loan on their house and started a software publishing business in their garage. Five years later, the business sold for $30 million.

He had built his training facility; had been shooting competitively for about 3 years; and, to this point, had been his own coach. He was shooting scores in the low 570s out of a possible 600 but needed to shoot in the mid-580s to make the national team. He thought that by working on his mental skills, he would gain the ground necessary to make the team.

Referral 6—Concentration Problems and Emotional Irritability

First Impressions

Initially, we wanted to know if there was a predictable pattern to Natasha's concentration problems and emotional irritability (e.g., coinciding with her menstrual cycle or directly relating to the level of stress within the competitive environment). Our next question was whether her coach was male or female.

Reasons for Our Questions

This was a 30-year-old female athlete, and the problems she described were not all that infrequent in menstruating females. Our second question arose from experiences we'd had with male coaches who were either genuinely insensitive to such problems or simply refused to acknowledge their existence.

We wanted to see whether there was any relationship between biochemical changes and performance or between stress and the breakdown in control. We certainly desired a better behavioral understanding of Natasha's use of the term "crazy."

Implications

If Natasha's menstrual cycle was making it more difficult for her to concentrate and to control emotions, then her problems would be greatly affected by the responses of others. A coach's response can be especially important. If the menstrual cycle is the issue, effective interventions must involve the coach and perhaps even teammates. We would want not only to test the athlete, but also to assess the attitudes and interpersonal skills of the coach.

Answers to Our Questions

A brief discussion with Natasha revealed that her concentration problems and emotionality were closely tied to her menstrual cycle and not to any particular environmental stressors. Her coach was male and, in the athlete's words, "not very empathetic." Natasha was concerned because her problems seemed more severe than those of her teammates and because she didn't like herself very much when she "behaved like a bitch." She had spoken to her gynecologist and was taking some medication that helped, but did not eliminate, the problem. Any suggestions we had about coping more effectively with the symptoms would be helpful.

Referral 7—Testing Prior to Olympic Trials

First Impressions

Based on the referral, we were left with several questions: What tests were used, and how were they helpful? Were these athletes in competition with one another for positions on the team? Had the coach, Oscar, discussed testing with the athletes?

Reasons for Our Questions

We asked about previous testing because when coaches have found something helpful, they often form very strong opinions about what they want or about how services should be delivered to the athletes.

If the athletes were competing with each other for positions, it would certainly affect their responses on any assessments. It would also affect how they would view our involvement and whether they would trust us.

The question about whether Oscar had discussed psychological testing with the athletes was important because athletes' cooperation depends on their attitudes towards testing and towards the service providers.

Implications

Whenever testing is introduced to a group of individuals, it is important to try to create a response set that will improve the likelihood of honest responses. When athletes are in a situation where important decisions have yet to be made about their competitive lives (e.g., whether they will be selected for a team or not), there will be some suspicion about testing and about how it will be used. Unless you minimize that suspicion, you are not likely to get the information you want. The answers to our questions would play a critical role in terms of how we would introduce testing and whether we would agree to get involved.

Answers to Our Questions

Oscar told us he had benefited from feedback about himself. He said that information from testing had helped him to understand and to communicate with the athletes he was working with at the time. He told us that he was willing to take the test again and that he didn't mind if his scores were shared with the athletes.

When I asked Oscar if the athletes knew he wanted them to take the test, he said no. He then told me, "It shouldn't matter to them. If they can't take a look at themselves, they've got problems. We are doing this for them." Oscar's words and behavior seemed to indicate that the athletes should be able to take any decision he made, on faith. If they couldn't, then they would have to shape up quickly or leave.

The athletes were competing with one another for spots on the team, and Oscar admitted that this was creating problems for him. Two of his best athletes were "playing mind games" with each other and were consistently competing for the coach's attention. They apparently disliked each other, and their inability to get along was affecting other athletes because they were talking "behind each other's back." They were also trying to persuade other athletes and individuals who weren't even involved with the team to take sides. Oscar's attempts to encourage the athletes to function in a more cooperative, team-oriented way were not working. He was hoping that our involvement and the testing would help him to confront the issues more effectively.

We told Oscar that we probably wouldn't get honest responses from the athletes unless they knew that the test results would be confidential and that nothing would be shared with anyone, including the coach, without the athletes' permission. The coach did not want to hear this and became angry: "How in the hell can I help the athletes if I don't know what is going on?" We talked about the issue at some length, and he finally, but reluctantly, agreed to allow us to keep the data confidential.

Referral 8—School Problems

First Impressions

This was a clinical issue; its resolution required family therapy and perhaps medication for Bobby. We weren't sure we wanted to be involved. If we did decide to get involved, we would need a very specific understanding of the problems the school was concerned about.

Reasons for Our Assumptions

Ten-year-old Bobby was probably controlling the relationship with his parents. His father was either unable or unwilling to be honest with his son, to confront him directly, or to set appropriate limits. The father was, in effect, asking us to participate in a lie. Our collective experience told us that the parents' inability to set limits was a primary contributor to Bobby's problems in school. Unless the parents could take more responsibility and earn Bobby's respect, our involvement wasn't likely to be very helpful.

Implications

We had to make a decision. First, did we want to involve ourselves in a clinical issue? If so, should we approach the problem as the father had suggested (i.e., from a sport psychology perspective) and gradually involve the family, or should we insist on treating it as a family issue from the start?

Answers to Our Questions

When we asked the father why he was allowing his son to refuse help, he told us that Bobby was very stubborn. The father knew from experience that if his son decided he didn't want to do something and someone "tried to force the issue, he would make life miserable for everyone." Rather than fight a losing battle, the father was hoping a more subtle and, admittedly, "sneaky" approach might work.

According to his father, Bobby was hyperactive. Though he had good perceptual and motor skills, he couldn't seem to stay focused on one task for any length of time. Concentration seemed to be much less of a problem for him in athletic situations, especially during competitions. In practice, Bobby frequently was disruptive but was responsive to the coach's discipline. In class, the problems were much worse. He was disruptive, and the teachers couldn't control him. He was having problems reading, and he refused to participate in many classroom activities. Attempts at discipline weren't having the desired effect. The father admitted that he had similar problems when he was in school but that he "eventually grew up."

Because the primary problems occurred at school and not in sports settings, we recommended that the father take Bobby to see a child-and-family counselor.

Referral 9—Driving Under the Influence

First Impressions

We had some questions: What were we expected to do for the athlete that wasn't already being done by the counselor? How committed was the coach to Dirk?

Reasons for Our Questions

The counseling that goes on between an Employee Assistant Program (EAP) worker and an athlete is confidential. We needed some idea of the coach's attitude toward that counseling. Did he think it was fulfilling its purpose (i.e., helping Dirk with his alcohol problem)? Was our role really going to be performance oriented, or did the coach also want us to monitor the alcohol issue? We have been in situations where coaches have not been that committed to athletes. Sometimes we were called in to help, but the real agenda had little to do with the athlete as a person. The real agenda in this case was to get enough information to make an immediate decision about whether to keep Dirk or to trade him.

Implications

If the coach was dissatisfied with the EAP worker and the progress she was making, knowing why would help us to define our role (e.g., performance focus, alcohol counseling, or both) and to determine how important it would be to work with the counselor.

When we get a referral, we want to define the issues clearly enough to provide a very specific focus for any testing and intervention. This means, as we have stressed, that we must translate the problem (e.g., "hasn't performed up to his potential") into concrete behaviors. What specific behaviors indicated Dirk was performing poorly? In what ways must his behaviors change? If the problem was still alcohol related and the coach was afraid the counseling wasn't working, why? What was it about Dirk's behavior or the overall situation that was generating the coach's concern? What would make the coach feel better about the situation?

Answers to Our Questions

The coach was committed to Dirk: "Dirk is the future of our team. I'd trade six other people before I'd get rid of him." The coach was concerned about the counseling. However, he wasn't concerned that the counselor wasn't capable; he was simply questioning whether or not the counseling was enough. He felt that the drinking problem was related to several other issues. Dirk was young, and away from home for the first time. He had money but was naïve in managing it. In addition, Dirk had not been performing as expected, and the coach believed the athlete's lack of confidence and his disappointment to be contributing factors. The coach wanted us to provide any information that would help the team to help Dirk. He wanted us to work on Dirk's concentration skills and his ability to control anger and frustration.

Summary and Conclusions

The initial reason given for seeing a sport psychologist is often vague because the coach or athlete is unable to adequately define the problem on his or her own. Your ability to operationalize a problem will enable you to

1. determine what tests, if any, to use;

2. identify the specific behaviors and environmental contingencies that affect the individual's ability to perform;

3. determine the specific steps to take in order to help the individual make critical decisions and perform at a higher level; and

4. convince your client that you know what you are talking about and motivate him or her to take the steps necessary for improvement.

Getting a clear understanding of the issues will require good analytical and conceptual skills. You must develop the habit of asking yourself and your client questions that will highlight any logical inconsistencies in the information they give you (e.g., "You are coming to me for help, but you don't have a problem?"). When a referral comes from someone other than the athlete concerned, you must put yourself in the position of both the athlete and the person making the referral, so you can gauge the nature of their interactions. What qualities of the person making the referral might be contributing to the identified problem? How will the interaction between the athlete and this person affect what you do?

Don't be afraid to admit that you don't understand the terms or descriptions used by the athlete or by the person making the referral. Encourage the individual to tell you, from a behavioral perspective, exactly what he or she means. Do not assume that you know. For example, if an athlete says, "I hate behaving like a bitch," what exactly does that mean? How does the individual want to behave? What specific behaviors must change and in what situations? An athlete may say, "I can't concentrate," but what does that mean? When does he or she have problems concentrating and what prevents that concentration? What happens to his or her concentration? Should the athlete be paying attention to something other than what he or she actually is paying attention to?

The interviewing and testing process is designed to help you zero in on critical issues—to obtain a clearer and clearer definition of the problem. After testing and an initial interview, you should have a good idea of

- the frequency of a problem (how often and in what different situations it occurs),

- the intensity of a problem (how long it takes and how difficult it is for the individual to control the problem once it occurs), and

- the specific conditions that increase or decrease the likelihood that the problem will recur.

It is absolutely critical that you take the time to behaviorally define the words and terms that others use and to look for logical inconsistencies in the referral. If you want a good exercise, go back over the referral questions (not our discussions of them) and see how many logical inconsistencies you can find.

When different pieces of information fit together as expected, you really don't learn anything new. When things don't fit neatly together, you may become confused, but you also have a unique opportunity to learn something integral to the case. Your ability to spot logical inconsistencies like the one below is the key to asking the kind of questions that will bring things into focus and into line.

You are a professional baseball player, playing in the World Series, and you're a choker? That doesn't make sense to me, at least not the way we define choker. You made an error, so what? You've made errors before. What's so different about this one?

Introducing Testing: Response Sets and Response Styles 5

You have decided to administer a psychological test because you believe it will add to your understanding of the person and provide the information you need to help the individual develop a mental-skills training program designed to enhance performance. What are the chances that the client's responses to the test will provide you with accurate information? To what extent will you have to use your own analytical skills to make mental adjustments in the elevation of test scores so that they more accurately represent the individual's actual skills and abilities?

Information gained from the assessment process is often used to make important decisions. These decisions can have a dramatic impact not just on the person tested but also on significant others (e.g., teammates and family members). It doesn't matter if you are using the test data to help in the development of a mental-skills training program or to aid in the selection process; you have a responsibility to ensure that the information is accurate. Can you possibly do that if you have never seen or spoken to the athlete?

You can't be sure that test information is accurate if you haven't had the opportunity to speak with the individual or to in some other way determine the effects that any response sets and response styles may have had on test scores.

A *response set* can be thought of as a situation-specific attitude that the athlete takes toward the testing process. This attitude can have a dramatic impact on the individual's willingness to cooperate with testing and on the way he or she responds to test items. *Faking* is a response set that some individuals adopt when they aren't sure how the information gained from testing will be used.

In contrast to a response set, a *response style* can be thought of as a more enduring, or cross-situational, personality characteristic. Like response sets, response styles influence how the individual responds to test items. You should be particularly sensitive to two response styles. The first is a dramatic or extreme response style, frequently seen in individuals who tend to adopt an extreme attitude toward situations. Behaviorally, these individuals often come across as dramatic; their language is packed with colorful adjectives. For them, life is a bit like a soap opera, and emotions can be fairly extreme.

The second type of response style is much more conservative. People with this style perceive everything in shades in gray. They think twice before they respond, and they tend to qualify everything: "Yes, I do that, but only when...." The language these individuals use to describe things is filled with qualifiers like "sometimes"; "at times"; "occasionally"; "yes, but"; "maybe"; and "you can't be sure."

To better understand the influence response sets and response styles can have on test scores, it is important to consider some actual data. Because we will be using scores from The Attentional and Interpersonal Style (TAIS) inventory, this is a good place to introduce you to the way scores are plotted on a profile sheet.

Figure 3 plots out the scores of the average world-record holder on 17 of the 20 TAIS scales. The percentile scores at the left of the graph are based on scores for the general population; thus, the average person in the general population would score at the 50th percentile on all 17 scales. The shaded area above each scale shows the range within which most world champions score on that particular characteristic. The dark line connecting various parts of the graph plots the profile of the average world champion. A brief definition of each scale is listed under the figure. As you will see later, there is a reason for the way we have connected certain scores.

Selecting a Comparison Group

Based on the scores shown in Figure 3, what conclusions can you draw about the average world-record holder? Consider the following:

- She has good concentration skills (BET relative to OET, BIT relative to OIT, NAR relative to RED).

- Her greatest concentration skill is focus. She is more focused and pays more attention to the little things than does 85% of the general population (NAR).

- She is highly competitive (P/O), willing to take responsibility (CON), and very confident (SES).

Do these statements have any real meaning? They do if you have a working knowledge of the concentration and interpersonal skills of the relevant groups. Here, you must know the skill level, in all areas, of the average person in the general population. You must also be aware of the average skill level of world-record holders. Knowing this will enable you to look at the abilities of the world-record holder and say, "Yes, the scores are accurate. Yes, the average world-record holder is more focused than 85% of the general population. Yes, the average world-record holder is more willing than 90% of the general population to take control and to assume the initiative. Yes, the average world-record holder is more confident than 80% of the general population."

When this particular subject responded to the items on the test, she mentally compared her skills to those of people familiar to her; this amounts to an implicit or an explicit response set. In the world-record holder's case, were those people average, or did she compare herself with other world-record holders? If, in the above case, she compared herself with the aver-

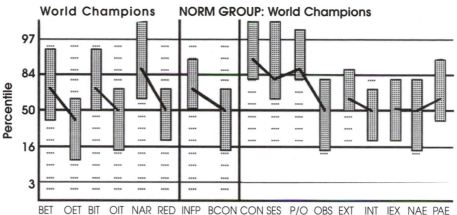

Figure 3. TAIS profile and scale descriptions.

BET: External awareness, or "street sense."

BIT: Analytical skill, strategic thinking, and problem solving.

NAR: Focus and follow-through, attention to details.

INFP: Information-processing capacity and need for change and diversity.

CON: Control/leadership, willingness to take responsibility.

P/O: Physical competitiveness, willingness to go "head to head."

EXT: Extroversion; enjoyment of, and need for, involvement with others.

IEX: Intellectual expression, willingness to express ideas in front of others.

PAE: Expression of positive feelings and willingness to support others.

OET: External distractibility.

OIT: Internal overload, tendency to become distracted by thoughts and feelings.

RED: Failure to shift from an external to an internal focus, or vice versa.

BCON: Impulsivity and/or nonconformity. High score is more impulsive.

SES: Self-esteem and self-confidence.

OBS: Speed of decision making. High score means slow decisions.

INT: Introversion; enjoyment of, and need for, personal space and privacy.

NAE: Expression of anger and willingness to confront and set limits on others.

DEP: Self-criticalness.

age person, she is an average world-record holder. If, on the other hand, she was mentally comparing herself with her competitors, she is an exceptional performer, even for a world-record holder.

Your skill as an interpreter of test information is directly related to

- your ability to determine with whom the individual has compared him- or herself and

- your knowledge of the skills and abilities of the athlete's comparison group relative to the group you wish to use for comparison.

Absolute Elevation and Relative Position of Test Scores

When you attempt to draw conclusions about an individual based on a set of test scores from an inventory measuring several different characteristics, you should look at the scores in two ways. From a training perspective, you should be most concerned with the relative position of test scores to one another, because you will want to use the information from testing to identify *relative* strengths and weaknesses. Even world-record holders can improve. By looking at relative strengths and weaknesses—even though a world-record holder's area of weakness may be considered a strength when compared to the average person's area of strength—you can focus on what needs the most work.

In a selection and screening situation, you should concern yourself with both the *relative position* and the *absolute elevation* of test scores. The relative position of scores (e.g., the person is more focused than analytical) tells you whether the individual is well suited to the demands of the sport or the job. The *absolute elevation* indicates how effective the person is in comparison to others: Person A scored at the 50th percentile on the scale measuring analytical skill, and Person B scored at the 80th percentile. In other words, the profile pattern gives you insight into an individual's strengths and weaknesses. The elevation of the profile helps you to predict the individual's performance relative to the comparison group.

When testing is used for training purposes, the relative position of test scores tends to be stable for most people. Additionally, training situations give you sufficient time to correct any mistakes in interpretation; this dramatically lowers the risk of making a decision that could harm the subject. Still, selection and screening situations place considerable pressure on people to respond in ways that may not reflect their actual abilities. Whenever there is a lack of trust or a doubt about how the information will be used, there is an increased risk that test information will be inaccurate.

Detecting the Influence of Response Sets and Response Styles

It is time for you to play detective again. Use your analytical skills to anticipate how various situations and attitudes might affect responses to an instrument like TAIS or to any other instrument you use. The specific items on your inventory and on the response choices the person makes will come into play. On TAIS, the respondent is limited to the following answers:

1. Never

2. Rarely

3. Sometimes

4. Frequently

5. Always

List some situations in which you think a person would be likely to *fake good*, or to at least minimize weaknesses and maximize strengths. Describe the specific effects these response sets would have on the relative position of scales to one another and on the absolute elevation of the profile.

_____

_____

_____

_____

List some situations that might encourage an individual to *fake bad*, or to exaggerate weaknesses. How would these response sets affect the absolute elevation of the profile and the relative position of scores?

_____

_____

_____

_____

Are you a person who is more than willing to share your thoughts and feelings with others? Do you see yourself as spontaneous and relatively uninhibited? If so, how would your style affect your test scores?

_____

_____

_____

_____

Are you a person who thinks carefully about things before making decisions? Do you work hard to avoid making mistakes? Do you try to see all sides of every issue? If so, how would your style affect your test scores?

_____

_____

_____

_____

Figure 4 shows the kind of profile typical of a subject who attempts to fake good on TAIS. You would expect to see profiles like this one most often in selection and screening situations. You might also see this when a subject is applying for a job, or any time an individual has something positive to gain by looking good.

The individual profiled in Figure 4 is the head of research and development at an international sports-marketing firm. His boss, the CEO of the organization, asked him to respond to TAIS, telling him that the information would be used for team-building purposes. What about this profile indicates that the person has not described himself accurately? We will give you a hint and tell you that most people taking a psychological test aren't sure

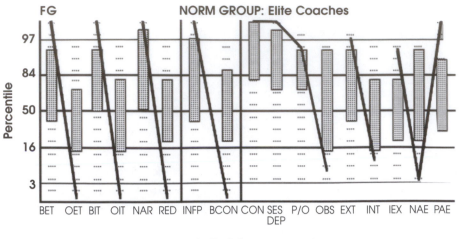

Figure 4. Faking good.

what is being measured. People taking TAIS usually don't know that the inventory measures 20 different concentration and interpersonal skills. They couldn't tell you the names of the different scales or which items fit which scales; even if they could, they would have a very difficult time (looking at items one at a time) figuring out how these items should fit together to create the perfect job profile. For these reasons, when people fake, their response set is fairly simple. They read an item and ask themselves, "Would it be good or bad to endorse this item?" It's almost an all-or-none response set. Now, how will that affect the absolute elevation and the relative positions of an individual's scores?

- Scales measuring what are perceived to be positive characteristics will be extremely high, and scales measuring what are perceived to be negative characteristics will be extremely low (e.g., above the 97th percentile and below the 3rd percentile respectively).

- There will be no differentiation between positive attentional scale scores (all will be at about the same height—BET vs. BIT vs. NAR), and there will be no differentiation between negative attentional scale scores (OET vs. OIT vs. RED).

There will also be many inconsistencies between the profile of someone faking good and what you know about the individual and about the demands of the job:

- The profile in Figure 4 suggests that if you gather 100 people in a room, the profiled individual would be more sensitive to the environment (BET) than everyone else, better at analyzing and planning (BIT), and superior at focusing and following through (NAR). The probability of this actually being the case is infinitesimal. Einstein might have been the most analytical, but he was far from being the most externally aware.

- The individual has indicated that he never makes a mistake due to becoming externally distracted (OET), internally distracted (OIT), or too narrowly focused (RED). The truth is, everyone makes mistakes.

- The individual has indicated that he is in control of every situation (CON), but that he expresses anger and/or confronts people and issues less often than does 97% of the general population (NAE). A person can't be in control that often without being somewhat confrontational.

These are general rules you can use to tell when a profile is invalid, either because the person faked or because the person has poor self-awareness. There are important differences between these two reasons, and you'll need to interview the person following testing to determine which is the case.

Although the scores in Figure 4 are like those you would obtain if someone faked, this particular individual insisted that he had not. His peers described him as talented, arrogant, egotistical, stubborn, and talkative. Not surprisingly, they also said he was a poor listener. He would dominate meetings and pontificate. He even behaved this way around his CEO. Given this information, how would you interpret his test scores? What conclusions can you draw about the accuracy of the interpersonal scores? What conclusions can you draw about the accuracy of the attentional scores?

On the interpersonal side, this individual's scores on the control (CON), self-esteem (SES), and intellectual expressiveness (IEX) scales certainly seem to be consistent with the descriptions provided by others. In addition, their description of him as egotistical and arrogant is consistent with the entire test profile. Here is an individual who sees himself as having no weaknesses. He is, in fact, quite talented, as we would expect the head of the research and development division of an international corporation to be. Unfortunately, he is also incredibly lacking in self-knowledge. This is perhaps his greatest flaw. He believes he has no problems, and he won't listen to anyone else; he is always right, and others are always wrong.

Clearly, the attentional scales do not accurately reflect this person's relative strengths and weaknesses. He isn't aware of them, so he can't tell you about them. How would you address these issues in a feedback session? How would you try to get him to listen to what you have to say? Providing

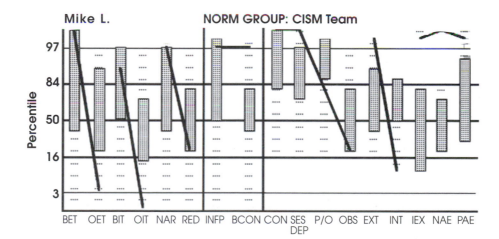

Figure 5. Navy SEAL. The shaded area on the profile shows where most (68%) of the individuals trying out for the team scored on each TAIS scale.

feedback to such an individual is something you will be required to do, and it's an exercise we will ask you to engage in later.

The individual whose profile is illustrated in Figure 5 is one of 15 U.S. Navy SEALs who had been invited to try out for a Navy pentathlon team. If selected, this individual would compete with four other SEALs against teams from all of the NATO nations. The competition comprises five events. Each individual competes as an individual in all events, and points are awarded for speed and accuracy. There is an individual winner (the individual with the highest point total) from all of the nations, as well as a winning team (combined score for the five members). Navy SEALs are typically chosen for the United States team because the events involve swimming, seamanship, marksmanship, running, and completing a complex obstacle course. This individual is a noncommissioned officer.

The commander of the group is an officer who has never competed in this type of event. His role is to oversee training and to get the team ready. He heard about TAIS and requested testing, indicating that the testing was to be used to provide feedback to individuals who were trying to make the team. He told his athletes, "I want the best team possible. This means that I want everyone to be able to perform to potential. Test information may be used to help each of you do just that."

After looking over Figure 5, consider the following questions regarding the Navy SEAL represented:

- What kind of response set did this individual have?

- How did his response set affect the absolute elevation of his scores?

- How did his response set affect the relative position of TAIS scales to one another?

- What in the profile is consistent with what you know about the individual's background and about Navy SEALs?

- What kind of problems might develop for this person in training prior to the competition?

- What kind of problems might occur during the competition?

- How would you behave when providing feedback to this person?

- What kind of behavior would you expect to observe during the interview?

TAIS inventory was administered before selection for the competition took place. Unfortunately, the competitors were not given a choice about responding to the inventory. Under such conditions, the competitors' respect for the commander and for the test administrator, combined with their level of trust in the reason for testing, was critical.

This Navy SEAL appears to have a rather dramatic response style. The extreme differences between scores suggest that he views the world as black or white. The profile pattern is not consistent with faking (e.g., very high BCON and NAE); indeed, this individual has made it a point to tell you that he is not afraid of anything. He obviously has a very high opinion of himself and his abilities. The scores that are most likely to be out of line in a case

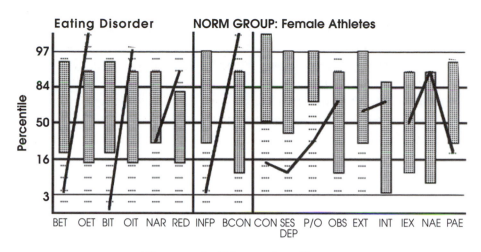

Figure 6. Olympic diver.

like this are the attentional scores because, like most people, our SEAL has not learned how to systematically evaluate concentration skills. He can see how extroverted or competitive or controlling others are, but the observable behaviors associated with having good analytical skills or the behaviors indicating distractibility aren't as obvious to him. It is doubtful that his attentional skills are as highly developed as he seems to believe they are.

Although the general profile pattern is consistent with that of the comparison group (CISM competitors who are SEALs), this individual's scores are still extreme. He takes pride in the fact that he does things his way (BCON). His scores on the expressiveness scales (IEX, NAE, and PAE) indicate that he keeps nothing back. He is going to do what he wants to do, whether you like it or not.

This individual challenges and confronts others. He can be intimidating, and he doesn't back down. He makes decisions very quickly (OBS) and acts on them. Although these attributes may be valuable in a combat situation, they are likely to get him into trouble the rest of the time. He is not a person who responds well to authority, yet he must respond to the chain of command in the military.

In the interview, he will quickly take control of the situation. He will begin to ask the questions, and he will tell you how it is. If you disagree with him, you will be wrong; and if you push too hard, you may begin to feel threatened.

Figure 6 represents a 20-year-old world-class diver who had been working with the same coach for the past 2 years. Her coach was selected to coach the Olympic team. This athlete not only had a good chance of qualifying for the team, but also a good shot at winning an Olympic medal. Testing took place approximately 6 weeks prior to the Olympic trials.

The coach gave the psychologist who administered the test a very warm introduction to the team. He explained that the results of testing would be used to provide feedback to the divers about their concentration skills, feedback that could be helpful to them as they attempted to make the Olympic team.

What kind of response set seems to be operating in this case? How would the response set affect the different scales on TAIS and the relative position of positive attentional characteristics (BET, BIT, NAR) to negative ones (OET,

OIT, RED)? Do you feel the absolute elevation of TAIS scores provides an accurate reflection of this young woman's current level of functioning? Is the relative position of her scores on the effective attentional scales (BET, BIT, NAR) consistent with high-level performance in the sport of diving?

Discussions with the coach about this diver prior to the administration of TAIS indicated that he did not see any major problems. From his perspective, she was extremely dedicated and hardworking. She was also very coachable and open to constructive feedback. According to the coach, her biggest weaknesses were being too hard on herself and being too much of a perfectionist. Considering this additional information, how accurate is the interpersonal side of her profile? How are you going to provide feedback to this young woman? How will you behave in the feedback session? What kinds of behavior do you expect to see on her part? Given a 2-year relationship with the coach and given the introduction the psychologist received, it is likely that this individual adopted a very open, self-disclosing response set. Knowing that the coach is unaware of any problems and that the diver is performing at a world-class level, it is doubtful that her scores reflect her actual behavior (e.g., what people observe). It would be difficult to perform as well as she currently performs and still have the high level of distractibility she has indicated. For this reason, you should question the absolute elevation of her test scores. The pattern of her scores, however, is consistent with the sport of diving. Her concentration strengths are her focus and follow-through (NAR). In closed-skill sports like diving, the tendency to become too narrowly focused (RED) and to ruminate and slow down decision making (OBS) can be a positive. High scores in those areas indicate a concern with being perfect and avoiding mistakes. In diving, the individual does not have to react quickly to another individual or to the environment. The diver can wait until he or she is ready to begin the dive. The high score on negative affect expression (NAE) is consistent with the coach's perception that this young athlete is too hard on herself.

The anomalies are the high distractibility scores (OET, OIT) and the low scores on the control and self-esteem scales (CON, SES). Given the conditions of administration in this case, the individual appears to be telling you more about how she is feeling about herself than about her actual performance. The test is providing an accurate description of her feelings, and she

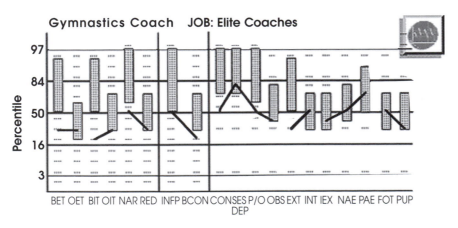

Figure 7. Women's gymnastics coach.

is asking for help. Keep this in mind when you come across similar inconsistencies with your clients.

In the interview, this woman admitted she was having serious problems controlling her bulimia. She would binge-eat and then panic at the thought of gaining weight. She was vomiting and was abusing drugs in an attempt to keep her weight under control. The coach was unaware of any of these problems.

Figure 7 represents a 30-year-old female and five-time world-champion gymnast who is now coaching at an Olympic level. The Gymnastics Federation mandated testing of coaches and athletes, but the athletes and coaches knew that the test information would be merely one additional piece of data used by the team psychologist to ensure that everyone was performing to potential. The psychologist had a long-standing relationship with the team and was trusted.

How do you think the conditions of administration might have affected the coach's scores? Is the profile consistent with the individual's history as you know it? What response style seems to be operating? Why is this profile more consistent with success in a sport like gymnastics than it would be with success in a team sport or in an open-skill sport like tennis or wrestling?

Whenever testing is mandated, it enhances the likelihood that an individual's responses to the inventory will be affected in ways that reduce the accuracy of the scores. In this instance, however, the coach's response style and her behavior in the interview suggested this was not the case. The pattern of the entire profile is consistent with the sport of gymnastics. The fact that all of the scores are in the narrow range, constricted but in a positive direction, suggests that this person is a perfectionist, someone who qualifies things and works hard to avoid mistakes. Her greatest strengths are her focus and her attention to detail (NAR). She is confident (SES) but willing to listen (CON is average); she is also positive (PAE).

In the interview, this woman came across as being quietly confident. She didn't have anything to prove; she knew what she had accomplished. She did more listening than talking, but she responded with assurance to any question dealing with her sport. She did not see herself as a technical instructor. In her mind, her role was to help prepare the athletes mentally for

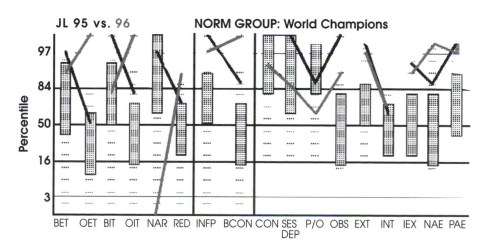

Figure 8. Response-set and response-style influences.

the competition. She believed she could do that, because she had been there and she knew what it took. Her quiet confidence seemed to rub off on her athletes. She was less effective when she had to deal with the politics of the federation; in those situations, she was not as assertive and confrontational as she needed to be.

Figure 8 shows two sets of TAIS scores for an individual who was the world's number-one ranked competitor (closed-skill sport) in 1995. Following her success in 1995, however, her ranking dropped to number three, and she began to struggle. She then referred herself to a psychologist for assistance. After a brief interview, she was asked to respond to TAIS using two response sets. First, she responded to the items as she believed she would have when she was ranked number one, in 1995 (black lines). Next, she responded to the items in a way that reflected how she was currently feeling about herself and her performance (red lines).

Independent of the two sets of scores, do you detect a more general response style? If so, what is it, and how will it affect the accuracy of the information you are considering? What was this woman motivated to communicate to the psychologist when she responded to TAIS?

Further discussions with the athlete provided the following information. After her quick rise to number one in 1995, she experienced some major life changes:

- She married another athlete who competed in the same sport;

- She began to draw serious attention from sponsors, promoters, and agents; and

- Her family, who hadn't paid much attention to her for years, began trying to take a more active role in her life.

Does this information affect your answers to the questions we asked about the athlete's response set? Does it affect your interpretation regarding the accuracy of the information?

We have presented this case for two reasons. First, an obvious response style affects her scores (and her actual behavior). Second, she was given a specific response set (e.g., first to answer TAIS items as they applied to her performance the year before, and then to answer them as they applied to her at the actual time of testing). In evaluating her and her issues, you need to keep both in mind.

The first profile, in which she refers back to 1995, suggests that this woman saw herself as being totally obsessed with her sport. She was feeling extremely confident and capable (CON, SES). Her TAIS scores show that she was easily distracted and could become too narrowly focused but that she obviously didn't care. The distractions and mistakes didn't matter, because she was feeling as if she was in control. She was successful in her chosen area (in her sport), and she was making mistakes in areas that didn't concern her. She was making them because her focus was on sport, and that was okay.

Her scores on both tests suggest a very dramatic response style. She lives life to the extreme, and it is very likely that her outward expressions are as dramatic as her test scores. In 1995, she was flying high and loving it. The changes she tried to dramatize in her responses regarding her feelings at the time of testing (in 1996) had to do with her having lost her single-mindedness. In her mind, she was completely unable to focus (NAR, OET, and OIT). She was not performing up to her potential and was becoming angrier and more emotionally impulsive (NAE, BCON).

It became obvious during the interview that she was delighted by all of the attention the media had given her. She was working hard to maximize the opportunities her success had created (e.g., endorsements, TV commentary) and she loved the attention. Given this, how do you think her extroversion and introversion (EXT, INT) will affect her ability to regain the number-one ranking?

Controlling Response Sets and Response Styles

How much should you try to control response sets and response styles by giving specific instructions prior to administering a psychological inventory? What do you stand to gain and what do you stand to lose when you manage an individual's responses? In which area would you be most interested in systematically controlling subjects' response sets: (a) research, (b) selection, (c) performance enhancement, or (d) team building? Why?

Traditionally, little has been done to control subject response sets during test administration. This is true independent of the reason for testing. If we create test items designed to evaluate your skills in a particular area (e.g., ability to focus concentration), with whom will you compare yourself? Will you evaluate your skills relative to those of your peers? Will you compare yourself with some ideal (e.g., the world's greatest performer, or perfection itself)? If the goal behind testing is to see if test scores will predict your level of performance, then it is in our best interest to make sure that when you respond to the inventory, you compare yourself with your competition. Not only that, but we will also want to provide you with anchor points that will give you an idea of how your average competitor would respond to the items. We might give the following instructions:

> We are trying to determine whether the inventory you are about to take can be used to accurately predict your performance relative to that of your peers in your sport. If it can, then we will be able to use the information we gain from the inventory to help people identify areas in which they may need work.

> As you respond to the items, respond as you believe they apply to you in your sport. Keep in mind that the average person you compete against would answer "sometimes" to most of the questions. If you are less easily distracted than most of your competitors, then that means you would respond with "rarely" or "never" to an item such as "I get distracted by my thoughts and feelings."

This instructional set might help to establish the validity of our inventory when it comes to predicting how well a person performs relative to peers in a research setting, where subjects are motivated to cooperate. It would not, however, be likely to influence subject responses in an actual selection and screening situation, particularly if the individual wanted to make the team and felt that test information might play some role in selection. Under those conditions, he or she would have a tendency to exaggerate strengths and to minimize weaknesses.

Even if subjects do adopt the desired response set, what information do we lose by controlling responses? When we insist that people compare their performance to that of their peers, we limit what we can learn about their true feelings and attitudes. Ask yourself how the profiles of the Olympic diver and the Olympic gymnastics coach would have looked if we had administered TAIS under such a response set.

With testing, individuals have an opportunity to tell you a great deal about their feelings; sometimes testing reveals as much or more about those feelings as it does about the person's actual performance. Both kinds of information are critical. Good coaching, good communication, and the maximization of performance depend as much upon an awareness of a person's feelings and attitudes as upon a person's actual skill level.

When testing, we allow subjects a good deal of freedom in determining how they will respond to questions. This places more responsibility on us to determine, after the fact, what their response set was. For us, the risk is worthwhile because we learn as much from response sets and styles as we do from the results of the inventory. Here is an example of the type of instructions we might give:

> The inventory we are asking you to respond to will provide us with information about your concentration skills and will tell us something about your interactions with others. This information will help us to understand you and to identify your areas of greatest strength and your areas of relative weakness. Please be as honest as you can in responding to the items.

Notice that we have not focused on any particular area (e.g., the sport), nor have we asked people to compare themselves with any particular group. Depending on the situation, we would add information to the above directive. In a selection situation, for example, we would tell the subjects that the information would be used as one part of a selection process, and we would emphasize that they are not required to respond to the inventory if they do not wish to do so. If they were going to receive feedback about the test, we would tell them. If we intended to share the information with others (e.g., a coach), we would get their permission. We would let them know that information would be treated confidentially, unless otherwise indicated.

Summary and Conclusions

Be aware of two different response styles. Think of behavior as falling along a dramatic versus cautious continuum. Most people tend to adjust their behavior along this continuum. There are, however, individuals who do not adjust their behavior to different situations; these are the individuals who fall at either end. Individuals with a dramatic style endorse the extremes on psychological inventories. Their behavior in interviews and in their day-to-day interactions with others mirrors this style. Some live life as if it were a soap opera, exaggerating everything. Individuals with a cautious response style behave in consistently moderate ways in their day-to-day interactions. They are slow to make decisions and slow to take risks. They are more concerned than most people about making a mistake. In contrast to the dramatic style, the cautious style gives people the appearance of being emotionally distant.

Although response styles help you anticipate and predict how an individual is likely to behave, they do not help you predict an individual's skill level (e.g., level of analytical skill compared with that of others). As a general rule, the dramatic person overestimates his or her abilities relative to those of others, and the conservative person underestimates them. When these response styles are operative, you must gather information from other sources (e.g., interviews, history) to accurately estimate the individual's level of competence relative to the competence of others.

Response sets tend to be situation-specific and can influence both the absolute elevation and the relative positions of scores. A response set is a temporary attitude, typically generated by the testing situation, that affects how a person answers test items. Some situations, like selection and screening, encourage individuals to try to look good. Other situations (such as seeking improvement) encourage individuals to exaggerate problems.

The instructions you provide for and the relationship you have with the individuals responding to the inventory will influence their responses. Your knowledge of each person, of the comparison group, of the demand characteristics of the situation, and of the constructs measured by the inventory—combined with your insight into how you would respond under similar circumstances—will allow you to evaluate the accuracy of the absolute elevation and relative position of an individual's scores.

Suggested Readings

Block, J. (1965). The challenge of response sets. In *Unconfounding meaning, acquiescence, and social desirability in the MMPI*. New York: Appleton-Century-Crofts.

Evens, J. (1989). *Bias in human reasoning: Causes and consequences*. Hillsdale, NJ: Erlbaum.

Assessment by the Numbers 6

Experienced test interpreters can do incredible things with test information. We have seen professionals draw accurate conclusions from TAIS scores in an uncanny manner. Lucky but educated guesses like, "I'll bet the guy is missing two fingers from his right hand" are almost too strange to believe. We've had people look at a TAIS profile and perfectly describe someone they had never met (but whom we know well). This level of skill takes time to develop. Where do you start?

The first step with any psychological test is to become familiar with the scales on the inventory. You already began this process relative to TAIS in chapter 3, when you were asked to provide behavioral examples of the different concentration skills and interpersonal characteristics measured by that inventory. Table 4 provides narrative descriptions of each TAIS scale, along with an indication of how the scale is to be interpreted.

Although you will require a thorough understanding of the individual TAIS scales, you don't want to rely too heavily on single scores when providing feedback. The richness of an individual's test results can only come out as you begin to look at the scores on the different scales in relationship to one another. In this chapter, we present a six-step process for interpreting TAIS results that involves looking at the relationships between scales. The steps are fairly simple. Your major challenge will be to interpret an individual's scores within the context of his or her sport. Your success in validating and effectively communicating test results will depend on your ability to link the scores to actual, performance-relevant behavior.

By the time you finish this chapter you should be able to

1. Write a one-paragraph description of an individual, based on TAIS scores, that captures the essence of the person—a paragraph that describes the individual's performance strengths, or the cognitive, personal, and interpersonal attributes that have contributed to the athlete's success up to the present time. You can then use this paragraph to begin your test feedback session.

2. Write a one-paragraph description, based on TAIS scores, that captures the kind of cognitive, personal, and interpersonal mistakes the individual is most likely to make as pressure increases. This information will help you explore possible problems in your feedback session with the athlete.

Table 4. The Attentional and Interpersonal Style (TAIS) Scales

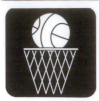

BET (Broad-External Awareness): The higher individuals score on this scale, the more capable they are of attending to a wide range of external cues. High scorers are good at assessing situations, reading nonverbal cues, and reacting instinctively to their environments. This "street sense" is important in many fast-moving, open-skill sports.

OET (Overloaded by External Information): High scorers make mistakes because they become distracted by task-irrelevant external cues. These individuals have a broad-external focus when it is inappropriate. For example, they fail to catch the ball because the movement of an opponent distracts them.

BIT (Broad-Internal Attention): High scorers are good at organizing and integrating a wide range of internal information (e.g., thoughts, ideas, feelings, and past experiences). These people are good at analyzing, planning, and using the past to anticipate the future. This attentional style is most important for developing strategies, analyzing opponents, and planning training programs.

OIT (Overloaded by Internal Information): High scorers make mistakes because they become distracted by their own thoughts at critical times. Their biggest mistake in sport is overanalyzing, either jumping to inappropriate conclusions (e.g., guessing a fastball when the pitcher throws a change-up) or failing to react because they are still thinking when they ought to be reacting.

NAR (Narrow/Focused): High scorers are good at narrowing their focus of attention, either externally or internally, as the situation demands. They are skilled at following through and at paying attention to details. They are perfectionists. Individual, closed-skill sports like golf, diving, and shooting, and sports that require a great deal of precision, place a heavy demand on this type of concentration.

RED (Reduced Flexibility): High scorers make mistakes because anxiety or anger interferes with their ability to make needed attentional shifts from an external focus to an internal focus or vice versa. Angry individuals become overly focused on the external sources of their anger and fail to think before acting. Anxious or worried individuals become overly focused on their own feelings and fail to react quickly enough to changes in the competitive situation.

INFP (Information Processing): High scorers on this scale become bored easily and need to be challenged mentally. They prefer a cognitively complex and continually changing environment. Low scorers are more comfortable, and perform better, in structured environments.

BCON (Behavior Control): High scorers are often seen as unconventional or impulsive (particularly by those who are more conservative). They tend to live by their own rules and to take more risks. They are more likely to compete in high-risk sports like downhill skiing. Low scorers tend to be more conservative, rule-bound, and in control of both their behavior and their emotional expressiveness (especially regarding anger).

CON (Need for Control): The higher individuals score on the control scale, the more they want to assume a leadership role and the more they feel as if they are in control of their lives. High scorers are more willing to take the initiative and to assume responsibility when leadership is lacking.

SES (Self-Esteem): High scorers on this scale describe themselves as competent and confident. Under pressure, the first emotion they feel is anger. Low scorers, on the other hand, react to pressure by becoming anxious and developing negative self-talk. This scale is positively correlated with the control scale. Thus, athletes who are in control tend to have high levels of self-esteem, while the opposite is true for those who are not in control.

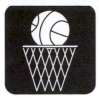

P/O (Physical Orientation/Competitiveness): High scorers have been physically competitive in the past and enjoy head-to-head competition with others.

OBS (Obsessive/Speed of Decision Making): This scale measures speed of decision making. A high scorer, someone who is "obsessive," tries hard to avoid errors and, as a result, considers every possible angle before making a decision. Low scorers on this scale make decisions quickly and move on. Differences between coaches and athletes in terms of their speed of decision making are a primary source of conflicts and breakdowns in communication.

EXT (Extroversion): High scorers on this scale need and enjoy socializing. They are outgoing and, when anxious, are likely to seek involvement with others. Not surprisingly, athletes involved in team sports tend to score higher on this scale than do athletes involved in individual sports.

INT (Introversion): High scorers enjoy personal space and privacy and may retreat from social involvement when under pressure. Among athletes who must room together, large differences in extroversion and introversion scores often create conflict.

IEX (Intellectual Expression): High scorers express their thoughts and ideas in front of others. They use their intellect and their verbal communication skills to solve problems and to motivate others.

NAE (Negative Affect Expression): High scorers are good at confronting issues and setting limits with people. They are not afraid to express criticism or anger. When this score is much higher than PAE, the individual is unlikely to be supportive of others when he or she is under pressure.

PAE (Positive Affect Expression): High scorers are supportive of and encouraging toward others. They need, and give, positive verbal and physical feedback (e.g., touching, patting). When NAE is very low, high scorers on the PAE scale may have difficulty setting limits on themselves and on others. Their desire to please others makes them susceptible to being taken advantage of.

DEP (Depression/Self-Criticalness): A high score is associated with being highly self-critical and with many of the feelings associated with depression (e.g., guilt and shame). Scores above the 90th percentile should serve as a warning that the individual's entire profile may be affected in negative ways. Because the DEP scale reflects feelings, scores will improve as the person's mood improves.

3. Use TAIS scores to generate testable hypotheses regarding the specific reasons for performance problems and to identify the specific steps needed to improve performance.

Predicting Performance

To accurately predict the conditions under which an individual will and will not perform well, it is important that you fulfill the following requirements:

- You must know about the athlete's technical and tactical skills and knowledge, and you must gather information about the technical and tactical demands of the performance situation.

- You must get information about the athlete's cognitive skills and abilities. For example, you must assess the person's ability to pay attention to the right things, to learn new information, to solve problems, to anticipate events, and to make good decisions.

- You have to assess the athlete's intrapersonal behavior to determine levels of drive and motivation, degree of competitiveness, willingness to take risks, and speed of decision making.

- You must assess the athlete's interpersonal behavior to gauge levels of extroversion, support, confrontation, and intellectual expressiveness.

- Finally, you need to determine how intellectually and emotionally stable the person is. To what extent can the individual keep anger, frustration, worry, or anxiety from interfering with the ability to make effective decisions and to perform?

TAIS Information

Information from TAIS will not tell you anything about the individual's technical and tactical skills or knowledge, nor will it tell you anything about the technical and tactical demands of the sport or the position. You must gather that information from other sources (e.g., from your own sports background, from the individual you are testing, from observations of performance, and from coaches). We have emphasized that you do not have to become a technical or tactical expert in every sport. You do, however, need two things:

1. You need enough knowledge about a particular sport to be able to draw upon sport-specific examples to illustrate the points you make when you are providing test feedback.

2. You need the input of a qualified expert in the sport to tell you whether or not the individual being tested has the technical and tactical talent and knowledge necessary for success. When there are technical and tactical weaknesses, you need to know what they are so that you don't automatically assume that the presenting problems are due to psychological factors.

Although TAIS does not measure the technical and tactical skills of an athlete or a coach, the instrument does provide information about the individual's cognitive abilities, intra- and interpersonal characteristics, and emotional stability. Table 5 shows you which TAIS scales are associated with different behavioral competency areas.

Table 5. TAIS Scale Loadings on Performance-Relevant Behavioral Competency Areas

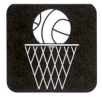

	TAIS scales
Technical/tactical skill and knowledge	——
Cognitive skills and abilities	BET, BIT, NAR, INFP
Personal attributes/intrapersonal skills	CON, SES, P/O, OBS
Interpersonal characteristics	EXT, INT, IEX, NAE, PAE
Emotional and intellectual stability	OET, OIT, RED, BCON, DEP

Presentation of Cases

In this chapter, you will be exposed to TAIS scores from six different subjects. Each case has been carefully selected to illustrate the diversity of issues you are likely to encounter when working with athletes. Because the cases involve different sports, the material will challenge you to develop enough understanding of each sport to be able to translate characteristics measured by TAIS into performance-relevant, sport-specific behavior. With each case, you will be provided the following information:

- the reason for referral,

- information about the athlete's technical and tactical skill,

- the conditions under which the TAIS was administered, and

- the individual's scores on TAIS.

This information will help you anticipate the subject's response set or attitude toward testing, and it will help you put TAIS results into a situational context. Because this is the first time a TAIS summary chart and profile have been presented together in this book, let's make sure you understand how the two relate.

Case 1 and the associated TAIS profile and summary chart present test scores for John, the elite sprinter we discussed in chapter 1. The summary chart at the top of the page lists John's scores alongside the average score for the comparison group on each of the 17 TAIS scales. John's scores are presented in the column labeled "You," and the average score for the comparison group is presented in the column labeled "Norm." In this example, the comparison group is male athletes (intercollegiate). As you can see by looking at the chart, John's score on the TAIS scale measuring external awareness, or BET, is at the 32nd percentile (compared with the general population). In comparison, the average male athlete scores at the 70th percentile (also compared with the general population).

Here is how to relate John's scores in the summary chart to his TAIS profile: The TAIS scale abbreviations on the profile (BET, OET, BIT, OIT, etc.) correspond to the brief scale descriptions provided in the summary chart. BET corresponds to John's score on the External Awareness scale; OET corresponds to John's score on the External Distractibility scale. Begin reading summary chart scores from the top left of the chart to the bottom right. Summary chart scores correspond to the scores on the profile when you read from left to right. Thus, the next-to-last score is Supportive/Encouraging, and the last score is Self-Critical. These two scores correspond to the PAE and the DEP scales on the profile.

When looking at a TAIS profile, keep the following in mind:

- The percentiles shown on the left side of the profile are based on the general population. Thus, the average person in the general population scores at the 50th percentile on every TAIS scale.

- The shaded area above each TAIS scale describes the area within which most of the individuals (68%) in the comparison group scored. For example, when it comes to the scale measuring "Need for Control/

Name: Sprinter   **Norms/Rating: Male Athletes**

Attentional Characteristics	You	Norms
External Awareness	32	70
External Distractibility	99	50
Analytical/Conceptual Skill	30	68
Internal Distractibility	80	50
Ability to Narrow Focus	88	60
Breakdown in Shifting Focus	99	55

Behavior Control		
Energy Need for Diversity	7	70
Impulsive/Nonconforming	70	60

Interpersonal Style		
Need for Control/Leadership	50	88
Self-Esteem/Confidence	17	83
Physically Competitive	98	90
Speed of Decisions/Worry	99	60

Interpersonal Style	You	Norms
Extroverted/Outgoing	15	75
Introverted/Private	93	45
Intellectually Competitive	10	45
Confrontive/Express Anger	2	50
Supportive/Encouraging	40	80
Self-Critical	99	35

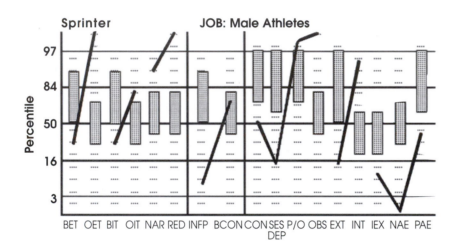

Leadership" (CON), 68% of the male athletes tested scored between the 75th and 97th percentiles.

- The black lines on the profile show where John scored on the different TAIS scales. The lines are connected so that they create a pattern or visual image you can use to quickly identify an individual's strengths and weaknesses.

- The test subject's score on the Self-Critical (DEP) scale is not plotted on the profile. To see how the person scored on the Self-Critical scale, you must look to the summary chart.

Why Some Plotted Scores Are Connected

The subject's scores on TAIS attentional scales are plotted on the profile sheet so you can immediately see the relationship between effective and ineffective concentration in three different areas. BET and OET are connected to one another because BET indicates the person has a broad-external focus of concentration when that is what the environment requires, and

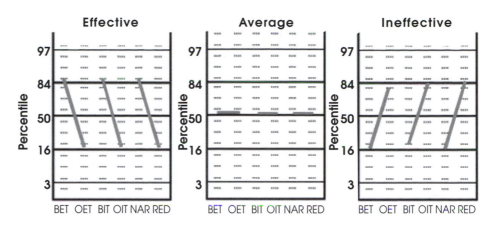

Figure 9. Patterns associated with various levels of concentration.

OET indicates a tendency to have a broad-external focus when it is not appropriate. BIT and OIT are connected because BIT indicates the likelihood that a person will have a broad-internal or analytical focus when that is required, and OIT indicates the likelihood that a person will have a broad-internal focus when he or she should not. Finally, NAR and RED are connected because NAR indicates the likelihood that the individual will narrow concentration when necessary, and RED indicates the likelihood that the individual will narrow concentration when it is not advisable. Figure 9 shows the patterns associated with highly effective concentration, average concentration, and highly ineffective concentration.

In addition to connecting effective and ineffective scores in the concentration areas, profiles are plotted to connect the individual's scores on the CON, SES, P/O, and OBS scales. These four scales can be thought of as intrapersonal characteristics, providing information about an individual's level of motivation, need to achieve, degree of competitiveness, and willingness to make decisions and take the initiative.

The subject's scores on the EXT and INT scales are also connected, as are scores on the three scales measuring expressiveness. These five scales measure important interpersonal characteristics. All of the connections are made to illustrate the importance of considering connected scores in relationship to each other when making your interpretations.

Six-Step TAIS Interpretation

Once you have all of the case-relevant information, you will be asked to use the following six interpretation steps to gather the information you need to describe the individual's performance strengths and weaknesses:

1. **Identify the individual's highest and lowest concentration scores** by comparing scores on the TAIS attentional scales measuring external awareness (BET), analytical skill (BIT), and focus and attention to detail (NAR). The highest attentional score represents the individual's concentration strength and indicates the skill the person will rely on under pressure. The lowest score indicates the concentration style the person will fail to shift to as pressure increases.

2. **Identify the individual's general level of competitiveness and willingness to take the initiative and to assume a leadership role** by looking at the average of his or her scores on the CON, SES, and P/O scales. How an individual scores on this cluster of scales indicates how that person will behave as pressure increases, and it allows you to predict the kinds of emotions (anger/frustration when scores are high vs. anxiety/worry when scores are low) most likely to interfere with performance.

3. **Identify the speed with which the individual makes decisions** by looking at the OBS score. The quicker the decision making (low score), the more willing the individual is to take a calculated risk and the more likely to make the mistake of reacting too quickly. A high scorer is a slower decision maker, more thoughtful and more concerned about avoiding errors altogether. High scorers usually make mistakes because they fail to react quickly enough.

4. **Identify the individual's level of comfort when interacting with others (EXT) and when working alone (INT).**

5. **Identify the individual's level of comfort when expressing ideas and feelings.** TAIS scores tell you how comfortable the person is with expressing thoughts and ideas (IEX); with challenging others, confronting issues, and expressing anger (NAE); and with expressing positive feelings, giving encouragement, and providing support (PAE). Which type of expression is the person most comfortable with, and which type is he or she least comfortable with?

6. **Identify the individual's level of cognitive and emotional stability** by looking at scores on the OET, OIT, RED, BCON, and DEP scales. Higher than average scores across these scales indicate less emotional stability and a greater likelihood that the individual will have problems performing well in pressure situations that require flexibility or "the ability to think and make adjustments on one's feet."

These are the six initial steps you will be asked to go through with each case before you attempt to describe the individual and his or her problem. We'll use John's TAIS scores as the first case and take you through the entire process. With the remaining cases, we'll expect you to work through the material and draw your own conclusions first.

Case 1—The Homesick Sprinter (Revisited)

Reason for Referral

John is a african-american sprinter at a predominantly White university in the South. He is participating in an elite-athlete development project and has been asked to respond to TAIS as part of that project. He knows that results from the inventory will be used to offer suggestions regarding specific steps he might take to improve his athletic performance.

As far as John's coach is concerned, John has all of the technical and tactical skill required to be a successful sprinter at a world-class level. The coach describes John in glowing terms and is extremely pleased with both his performance and his attitude. He is unable to identify any specific areas in which he thinks John might work to improve his performance.

Most Likely Response Set

We would expect John to be cooperative and relatively nondefensive. If he were highly motivated to be better, he might have a slight tendency to exaggerate some of his weaknesses, to point out problems he believes he has.

Technical and Tactical Skills

John's coach, who is highly regarded by other sprint coaches in the country, has indicated that John does have the technical and tactical skills required. We have no reason to doubt this.

Interpretation Steps

Concentration Strength and Relative Weakness

John is very good at focusing his attention, at following through and paying attention to detail (NAR). In sprinting, this type of concentration will help him focus at the start of the race and will ensure that he practices and perfects things such as his start and his baton-passing in relay races.

John's scores on both broad-external (BET) and broad-internal (BIT) are relatively low. His lowest score, however, is on broad-internal. Under pressure, he is not likely to make the mistake of overanalyzing. That's a plus for a sprinter. As a student, John may have difficulty with timed tests that require complex analysis (e.g., essay tests). When he has problems performing, he may also have difficulty getting at the cause on his own because of his relatively low score in the analytical area.

Confidence, Competitiveness, and Willingness to Take Control

John's score on the control scale (CON) is average for the general population, but relatively low for male athletes. He is extremely competitive (P/O), even for athletes. His level of self-confidence (SES) is quite low, but much of that can be attributed to the fact that the plotted self-esteem score takes into account a very high depression (DEP), or self-critical, score.

Because John's performance on the track is exceptional (according to his coach), it is likely that his depression and low level of self-confidence reflect his feelings when he is not training or competing.

Decision Making

John is very slow when it comes to making decisions (OBS). His score, especially when combined with a high NAR score, suggests he is a perfectionist. He tries to avoid mistakes at all costs. Because sprinting does not require complex problem solving and rapid decision making, this score should not create problems on the track; indeed, his perfectionism suggests he will work and train very hard.

Extroversion/Introversion

John is extremely introverted (INT), and he is much more comfortable when he is alone or with one or two people than he is when he has to socialize (EXT). This will make it harder for him to fit in with the team away from the track.

Emotional and Intellectual Expression

John is not very expressive. His highest score in the expressiveness area is on the scale reflecting the expression of positive feelings and support (PAE). On the PAE scale, John scores at the 40th percentile. John does not outwardly express anger (NAE) or many of his thoughts or ideas (IEX). If he says anything at all, it is positive. This pattern of scores undoubtedly contributes to his coach's impression that he is easy to coach.

Control Over Thoughts and Feelings

John's scores on the external (OET) and internal (OIT) distractibility scales indicate that he loses control over his thoughts quite easily. This is emphasized by a low score on the information-processing scale (INFP). John's elevated score on the reduced focus scale (RED) and moderately elevated score on the behavior control scale (BCON) suggest he also loses control over his feelings. The fact that negative affect expression (NAE) is so low, however, suggests that worry, anxiety, and self-doubt (SES) are more serious contributors to his distraction than anger. Indeed, John undoubtedly focuses any anger that he feels on himself (contributing to his depression and relatively low feelings of self-worth), rather than on someone else.

Performance Strengths

John is a highly focused, hardworking, dedicated athlete (NAR). He gets to practice on time and takes seriously everything the coach says. When it comes to track, he is extremely competitive (P/O) and a perfectionist (OBS). Quiet and introverted (IEX, INT), John is much more of a listener than a talker. He takes a good deal of time to think things over before making a decision. When he does speak, it's almost always in a positive, supportive way (PAE).

Most Likely Performance Error(s) Under Pressure

As pressure increases, John is likely to become too narrowly focused. His concern about avoiding mistakes (OBS) can lead to worry and self-doubt (RED, SES, and DEP). If that happens, John's introversion (INT) takes over, and he becomes very quiet, keeping thoughts and feelings to himself (IEX, NAE) and withdrawing from others. This behavior can keep him from getting the support he needs to work through issues.

Because John is so competitive and talented within the track environment (P/O), he is much more likely to have problems in other performance arenas—in school, for example. His low scores on the TAIS scales measuring analytical thinking (BIT) and intellectual expression (IEX), combined with a low self-esteem score (SES), suggest that he may be worried about academics.

Contributing Factors and Steps for Improvement

John's introversion causes him to withdraw from others even when he could use their support and help (INT). His lack of confidence in his ability to express himself contributes to that withdrawal, as does his extreme unwillingness to confront issues or to express any frustration, unhappiness, or anger (IEX, NAE).

Though John's narrow focus of concentration (NAR) is to his advantage in his sport, as pressure increases that focus makes it very difficult for him to broaden his perspective, either to bring in new information from the environment (BET) or to engage in good strategic thinking and problem solving (BIT). John's solution to problems is to withdraw.

CHAPTER 6

Given the fairly extreme nature of John's scores, it is unlikely that his behavior is going to change significantly without outside help. John will need the support and encouragement of others to get him to open up and express his thoughts and feelings. If academic concerns and pressures are contributing to John's unhappiness, he may benefit from stress management training, tutoring, and a course designed to teach him how to study and prepare for tests.

Lessons to Be Learned From Case 1

There are two important lessons to be learned from this case. The first is that it can be a mistake to assume that quiet, outwardly positive athletes are happy. It is not unusual to find athletes like John who lack confidence in their ability to express their thoughts and ideas (low BIT and IEX) and are uncomfortable when they have to do so. If these individuals become anxious (high RED and OBS) and depressed (DEP), they try to cope with problems by avoidance, withdrawal, or physical escape. For them, the easiest way to avoid an uncomfortable situation (e.g., one in which they are being asked for an opinion) is to agree with the other person. Most of the time, this is what is going on with individuals who appear to be doing well and then drop out of programs unexpectedly. Remember this score pattern for future reference.

The second lesson is that the characteristics that serve John well in one performance arena can really hurt him in another. As a student-athlete, John is required to perform in the classroom as well as on the track. His narrow focus (NAR), obsession with detail (OBS), lack of intellectual expression (IEX), and low score on the analytical scale on TAIS (BIT) can work for him in a sport where he has no time to think. Those characteristics, however, don't help him in the classroom.

When interpreting data, do not assume that your interpretations are correct. We've developed a number of hypotheses about John's ability to perform, based on the referral information and his TAIS data. We have confidence in TAIS, and we have confidence in our ability to interpret the inventory; but despite this confidence, it would be inappropriate to assume that all of our hypotheses are correct.

You are being asked to follow a particular format for analyzing TAIS results because this format will help you generate hypotheses about behavior that contributes both to the individual's success and to his or her failure. In the feedback interview, you will be asked to consensually validate or invalidate your hypotheses. You will then make recommendations based on the accuracy of your interpretations and the willingness of the subject to respond to your suggestions.

Case 2—An Olympic Hopeful (Revisited)

Reason for Referral

Pete is a highly successful entrepreneur, having just sold his business for $30 million. He sold his business so he could finance his dream of becoming an Olympic shooter. He is 42 years old and has been shooting competitively for 3 years. He is currently shooting scores between 565 and 570 out of 600. To make an Olympic team, he will need to consistently shoot around 585.

Name: Shooter　　　　**Norms/Rating: Closed Skill Champs**

Attentional Characteristics	You	Norms
External Awareness	80	55
External Distractibility	2	40
Analytical/Conceptual Skill	90	55
Internal Distractibility	20	27
Ability to Narrow Focus	90	83
Breakdown in Shifting Focus	22	55

Behavior Control		
Energy Need for Diversity	88	60
Impulsive/Nonconforming	5	40

Interpersonal Style		
Need for Control/Leadership	95	88
Self-Esteem/Confidence	99	68
Physically Competitive	83	78
Speed of Decisions/Worry	22	73

Interpersonal Style	You	Norms
Extroverted/Outgoing	70	50
Introverted/Private	75	60
Intellectually Competitive	83	50
Confrontive/Express Anger	2	50
Supportive/Encouraging	80	65
Self-Critical	2	35

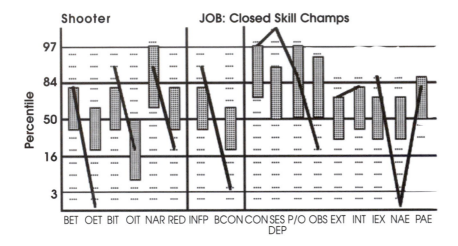

Pete has referred himself to you for help. He realizes that shooting is as much a mental game as it is a physical one. Before coming to you, he did a lot of research trying to find the best person he could. You came highly recommended.

What is the athlete's most likely response set?

_____

_____

_____

_____

Does the athlete have the technical and tactical skill required to be successful?

_____

_____

_____

_____

Interpretation Steps

What is the athlete's concentration strength and relative weakness?

_____

_____

_____

_____

How confident, competitive, and willing to take control is the athlete?

_____

_____

_____

_____

How quickly does the athlete make decisions?

_____

_____

_____

_____

Is the athlete extroverted, introverted, both, or neither?

_____

_____

_____

_____

How expressive is the athlete of thoughts, ideas, and feelings?

_____

_____

_____

_____

How easily does the athlete lose control over thoughts and feelings?

_____

_____

_____

_____

Describe the athlete's strengths within the context of his performance environment.

_____

_____

_____

_____

Describe the athlete's most likely performance error under increasing pressure.

_____

_____

_____

_____

What attentional and interpersonal factors contribute to the performance problem, and what steps can be taken by the athlete to improve?

_____

_____

_____

_____

What are the lessons to be learned from this case?

_____

_____

_____

_____

Case 3—Water Polo Madness

Reason for Referral

Howard is an extremely talented water polo player who can't seem to control his anger in pressure situations. According to his coach, Howard is without question the most naturally gifted athlete on his team, with the physical talent to be a real force in international competition. Unfortunately, Howard's anger and competitive intensity get the better of him, and he has developed a reputation for being a "head case." When he or his team doesn't perform up to his expectations, he becomes so angry and frustrated that he stops thinking, loses his touch, and tries to do everything himself. His passes are too hard, his shots are wild, and he tries to swim right through the opposition. Howard has come to you under the threat of being dropped from the team.

Name: Howard F.　　　　　　**Norms/Rating: Male Athletes**

Attentional Characteristics	You	Norms
External Awareness	88	70
External Distractibility	90	50
Analytical/Conceptual Skill	93	68
Internal Distractibility	99	50
Ability to Narrow Focus	1	60
Breakdown in Shifting Focus	55	55

Behavior Control	You	Norms
Energy Need for Diversity	95	70
Impulsive/Nonconforming	93	60

Interpersonal Style	You	Norms
Need for Control/Leadership	99	88
Self-Esteem/Confidence	83	83
Physically Competitive	95	90
Speed of Decisions/Worry	35	60

Interpersonal Style	You	Norms
Extroverted/Outgoing	65	75
Introverted/Private	60	45
Intellectually Competitive	98	45
Confrontive/Express Anger	93	50
Supportive/Encouraging	12	80
Self-Critical	50	35

Howard F.　　　　　　**JOB: Male Athletes**

Percentile

97
84
50
16
3

BET OET BIT OIT NAR RED INFP BCON CON SES P/O OBS EXT INT IEX NAE PAE
DEP

What is the athlete's most likely response set?

_____

_____

_____

_____

Does the athlete have the technical and tactical skill required to be successful?

_____

_____

_____

_____

Interpretation Steps

What is the athlete's concentration strength and relative weakness?

_____

_____

_____

_____

How confident, competitive, and willing to take control is the athlete?

_____

_____

_____

_____

How quickly does the athlete make decisions?

_____

_____

_____

_____

Is the athlete extroverted, introverted, both, or neither?

_____

_____

_____

_____

How expressive is the athlete of thoughts, ideas, and feelings?

_____

_____

_____

_____

How easily does the athlete lose control over thoughts and feelings?

_____

_____

_____

_____

Describe the athlete's strengths within the context of his performance environment.

_____

_____

_____

_____

Describe the athlete's most likely performance error under increasing pressure.

_____

_____

_____

_____

What attentional and interpersonal factors contribute to the performance problem, and what steps can be taken by the athlete to improve?

_____

_____

_____

_____

What are the lessons to be learned from this case?

_____

_____

_____

_____

Case 4—Gymnastics Superstar

Reason for Referral

Ludmilla is an Olympic champion and two-time world champion on the uneven parallel bars. An odds-on favorite to repeat in the upcoming Olympics, she was tested along with other Olympic hopefuls at a training camp approximately 3 weeks before the Olympic team was to be named.

The coach, in providing his impressions of all of the athletes prior to testing, indicated that Ludmilla is still a mystery to him. In spite of having been Ludmilla's coach for 10 years, he still cannot "read her" and does not know what motivates her or how she reacts to the things he says.

Testing was introduced to the entire team by the coach. He explained to them that the inventory measured concentration skills that are very important to performance. The purpose of testing was to provide each athlete with feedback about concentration skills, feedback that would help ensure performance up to full potential during competition. The athletes understood

TAIS PERCENTILE SCORES

Name: Ludmilla   **Norms/Rating: World Champs**

Attentional Characteristics	You	Norms
External Awareness	80	55
External Distractibility	50	40
Analytical/Conceptual Skill	40	55
Internal Distractibility	55	27
Ability to Narrow Focus	83	85
Breakdown in Shifting Focus	83	50

Behavior Control	You	Norms
Energy Need for Diversity	25	65
Impulsive/Nonconforming	50	40

Interpersonal Style	You	Norms
Need for Control/Leadership	88	88
Self-Esteem/Confidence	50	83
Physically Competitive	78	88
Speed of Decisions/Worry	90	60

Interpersonal Style	You	Norms
Extroverted/Outgoing	65	60
Introverted/Private	75	50
Intellectually Competitive	5	50
Confrontive/Express Anger	7	55
Supportive/Encouraging	30	73
Self-Critical	78	35

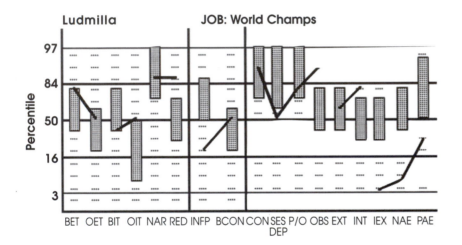

that information from testing would not be shared with the coach unless they gave permission.

What is the athlete's most likely response set?

_____

_____

_____

_____

Does the athlete have the technical and tactical skill required to be successful?

_____

_____

_____

_____

Interpretation Steps

What is athlete's concentration strength and relative weakness?

_____

_____

_____

_____

How confident, competitive, and willing to take control is the athlete?

_____

_____

_____

_____

How quickly does the athlete make decisions?

_____

_____

_____

_____

Is the athlete extroverted, introverted, both, or neither?

_____

_____

_____

_____

How expressive is the athlete of thoughts, ideas, and feelings?

_____

_____

_____

_____

How easily does the athlete lose control over thoughts and feelings?

_____

_____

_____

_____

Describe the athlete's strengths within the context of her performance environment.

_____

_____

_____

_____

Describe the athlete's most likely performance error under increasing pressure.

_____

_____

_____

_____

What attentional and interpersonal factors contribute to the performance problem, and what steps can be taken by the athlete to improve?

_____

_____

_____

_____

What are the lessons to be learned from this case?

_____

_____

_____

_____

Case 5—Life on the Edge

Reason for Referral

Heidi is a very talented speed skier with a history of career-threatening injuries. Her coach describes her as extremely difficult to work with. When things are going well, Heidi is on top of the world; when things aren't going well, she is almost impossible to tolerate.

Recently injured, Heidi agreed to respond to TAIS for two reasons. First, her coach had requested it, indicating that he wanted to understand her a little better and that he hoped it would help the two of them communicate. Second, Heidi herself was interested in anything she could do to recover more quickly from her injury and to prevent injuries in the future.

What is the athlete's most likely response set?

_____

Name: Skiing-Downhill   **Norms/Rating: Female Champions**

Attentional Characteristics	You	Norms
External Awareness	95	55
External Distractibility	20	45
Analytical/Conceptual Skill	75	55
Internal Distractibility	45	35
Ability to Narrow Focus	88	78
Breakdown in Shifting Focus	45	50

Behavior Control	You	Norms
Energy Need for Diversity	88	65
Impulsive/Nonconforming	70	40

Interpersonal Style	You	Norms
Need for Control/Leadership	99	85
Self-Esteem/Confidence	93	73
Physically Competitive	95	88
Speed of Decisions/Worry	35	60

Interpersonal Style	You	Norms
Extroverted/Outgoing	90	50
Introverted/Private	17	60
Intellectually Competitive	45	50
Confrontive/Express Anger	99	55
Supportive/Encouraging	95	73
Self-Critical	7	50

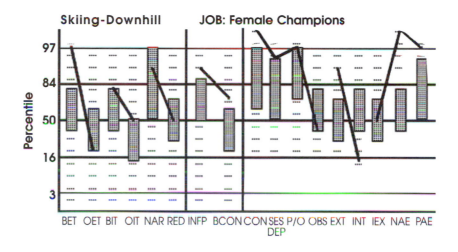

Skiing-Downhill   JOB: Female Champions

_____

_____

_____

Does the athlete have the technical and tactical skill required to be successful?

_____

_____

_____

_____

Interpretation Steps

What is the athlete's concentration strength and relative weakness?

_____

_____

_____

_____

How confident, competitive, and willing to take control is the athlete?

_____

_____

_____

_____

How quickly does the athlete make decisions?

_____

_____

_____

_____

Is the athlete extroverted, introverted, both, or neither?

_____

_____

_____

_____

How expressive is the athlete of thoughts, ideas, and feelings?

_____

_____

_____

_____

How easily does the athlete lose control over thoughts and feelings?

_____

_____

_____

_____

Describe the athlete's strengths within the context of her performance environment.

_____

_____

_____

_____

Describe the athlete's most likely performance error under increasing pressure.

_____

_____

_____

_____

What attentional and interpersonal factors contribute to the performance problem, and what steps can be taken by the athlete to improve?

_____

_____

_____

_____

What are the lessons to be learned from this case?

_____

_____

_____

_____

Case 6—The Moody Striker

Reason for Referral

Sarah is a talented striker on her college soccer team. She has been voted the most valuable player in the league for the past 2 years. Very bright and always looking for a competitive edge, she has come to ask you for help. She has noticed that just prior to the onset of menstruation, she has difficulty concentrating and feels less energetic than she does at other times. In spite of these feelings, Sarah's talent and mental toughness usually carry her through. Often she believes her feelings prior to menstruation cause more problems for her teammates than they do for her. She has agreed to respond to TAIS under two different response sets, hoping the information the inventory provides will help her and the team.

The dark lines on the profile and the percentile numbers under the "You" heading on the summary chart show Sarah's scores when she is feeling good (midcycle). The lighter lines on the profile and the percentile numbers under the "Norms" heading on the summary chart show Sarah's scores just prior to menstruation.

What is the athlete's most likely response set?

_____

_____

TAIS PERCENTILE SCORES

Name: Mid Cycle   **Norms/Rating: Pre Menstrual**

Attentional Characteristics	You	Norms	*Interpersonal Style*	You	Norms
External Awareness	80	32	Extroverted/Outgoing	70	50
External Distractibility	5	55	Introverted/Private	22	22
Analytical/Conceptual Skill	93	83	Intellectually Competitive	95	50
Internal Distractibility	27	27	Confrontive/Express Anger	32	55
			Supportive/Encouraging	73	55
Ability to Narrow Focus	99	60	Self-Critical	12	78
Breakdown in Shifting Focus	35	55			

Behavior Control	You	Norms
Energy Need for Diversity	95	80
Impulsive/Nonconforming	25	25

Interpersonal Style	You	Norms
Need for Control/Leadership	85	22
Self-Esteem/Confidence	99	98
Physically Competitive	95	60
Speed of Decisions/Worry	60	60

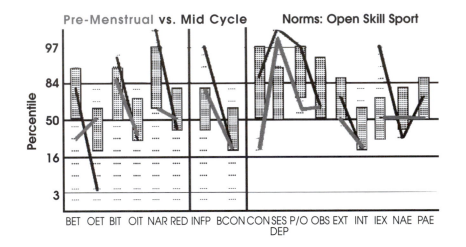

Pre-Menstrual **vs. Mid Cycle**   **Norms: Open Skill Sport**

_____

_____

Does the athlete have the technical and tactical skill required to be successful?

_____

_____

_____

_____

Interpretation Steps

What is the athlete's concentration strength and relative weakness (mid-cycle vs. premenstrual)?

_____

_____

How confident, competitive, and willing to take control is the athlete (midcycle vs. premenstrual)?

_____

_____

_____

_____

How quickly does the athlete make decisions (midcycle vs. premenstrual)?

_____

_____

_____

Is the athlete extroverted, introverted, both, or neither (midcycle vs. premenstrual)?

_____

_____

_____

_____

How expressive is the athlete of thoughts, ideas, and feelings (midcycle vs. premenstrual)?

_____

_____

_____

_____

How easily does the athlete lose control over thoughts and feelings (midcycle vs. premenstrual)?

_____

_____

_____

_____

Describe the athlete's strengths within the context of her performance environment (midcycle only).

_____

Describe the athlete's most likely performance error under increasing pressure (premenstrual only).

_____

_____

_____

_____

What attentional and interpersonal factors contribute to the performance problem, and what steps can be taken by the athlete to improve?

_____

_____

_____

_____

What are the lessons to be learned from this case?

_____

_____

_____

_____

Our Analyses
Case 2—An Olympic Hopeful

Reason for Referral (Recap)

Pete is the highly successful entrepreneur trying to become an Olympic shooter.

What is the athlete's most likely response set?
Because he is self-referred and has confidence in our ability to help, he will respond in a very open and honest way. We would expect very little distortion in test scores.

Does the athlete have the technical and tactical skill required to be successful?
We are not sure if he has the technical and tactical skill or the physical talent required to achieve his goal. We suspect that improving one's shooting score from 570 to 585 is much more difficult than improving from 555 to 570. Pete is relatively old. How long can shooters shoot high scores? We need more information.

Interpretation Steps

What is the athlete's concentration strength and relative weakness?
Pete has excellent concentration skills. He scored at the 90th percentile on both the scale measuring his analytical skill (BIT) and the scale measuring his ability to focus (NAR). His lowest score is on the external awareness scale (BET).

How confident, competitive, and willing to take control is the athlete?
Pete is very confident (SES), has a very strong need for control (CON), and is highly competitive (P/O). His scores in these areas are even higher than those of world champions in closed-skill sports (normative population).

How quickly does the athlete make decisions?
Pete has described himself as a moderately quick decision maker (low OBS), especially in comparison to the average score for world champions in closed-skill sports.

Is the athlete extroverted, introverted, both, or neither?
Pete's scores on both the extroversion (EXT) and introversion (INT) scales are relatively high, indicating he enjoys people but also enjoys his personal space. Given his high scores on the control scale (CON) and the self-esteem scale (SES), he will behave in an extroverted or introverted way on his own terms (e.g., when he wants to, as opposed to when others want him to behave one way or the other).

How expressive is the athlete of thoughts, Ideas, and feelings?
Pete indicates that he is more than willing to express his thoughts and ideas. His relatively high score on the IEX scale shows that he enjoys competing intellectually as well as physically. He describes himself as very positive and supportive (PAE): "The glass is always half full." He seems not to express anger or frustration (NAE).

How easily does the athlete lose control over thoughts and feelings?
Pete is highly controlled behaviorally (BCON) and keeps a tight rein on any feelings of anger (NAE). He makes very few concentration errors (OET, OIT, and RED). When he does become distracted, it is more likely to be a result of his own thoughts and feelings rather than of any external stimuli.

Describe the athlete's strengths within the context of his performance environment.
Pete has the ability to narrow his focus of concentration, to pay attention to details, and to follow through (NAR). These are characteristics of world champions in closed-skill sports. He is more than willing to take responsibility for his training (CON) and is extremely positive (PAE) and confident in his ability to succeed (SES). When it comes to establishing long-term goals and developing a training program designed to lead to the accomplishment of those goals, Pete has what it takes (BIT, NAR).

Describe the athlete's most likely performance error under increasing pressure.
As pressure increases, Pete will have at least two problems. First, his high scores on analytical skill (BIT), intellectual expressiveness (IEX), and information

processing (INFP) suggest that he will overanalyze and overcomplicate his situation. He will have too many ideas and lose the narrow focus required to perfect his shooting skills. Second, Pete's high scores on self-confidence (SES) and need for control (CON) indicate he will have difficulty trusting and respecting the skills and abilities of others. Under pressure, he will have confidence in his own analyses over those from any coaches or sport psychologists.

What attentional and interpersonal factors contribute to the performance problem, and what steps can be taken by the athlete to improve?
Practicing shooting can be extremely boring for an individual like Pete (INFP). His challenge is to develop a shooting routine and to practice, practice, practice. Practice requires focused, high-quality concentration. Pete will become bored and will constantly analyze his shooting (BIT); this ongoing analysis will lead him to experiment continually with everything from how he raises his pistol to what kind of grip to have to how to load his ammunition. Playing with these distractions will prevent him from focusing the way he must in order to shoot 585.

Pete's strong positive attitude (PAE) and high need for control will lead him to discount criticism from others (e.g., criticism for analyzing too much or for not sticking to the basics). Given both his respect for us at the beginning of the relationship and his positive attitude, Pete will agree with anything we say, provided it is sensible and logical. He will begin to disagree, however, as soon as he encounters problems in carrying out our suggestions. We may be able to help him stay on track by predicting potential problems. Also, Pete is so competitive, positive, and confident that we may be able to use these characteristics to get him to focus. We can do this by predicting that he will fail to accomplish his goal:

> *Pete, you are so analytical that you would be a much better coach than a shooter. We don't believe you can shut off your analytical thinking as much as you need to, to be successful. Shooting isn't rocket science. You raise the pistol and pull the trigger. We can give you procedures to use to help you temporarily let go of some of the analytical thinking so you can just focus on the shooting. These procedures, however, are as simple and straightforward as the shooting. To get them to work, you have to practice them over and over and over.*

What are the lessons to be learned from this case?
Here are some of the specifics you should take away from Pete's TAIS profile. These points will be applicable to many of the athletes you will work with in the future:

- High scores on the analytical scale (BIT) and the intellectual expressiveness scale (IEX) can create major problems for elite-level athletes, especially in sports where the individual must react quickly and instinctively to the situation. Coaches talk about "paralysis by analysis," and this is what you are likely to get from athletes with high BIT and IEX scores, especially if they are competing in sports that demand instinctive responses (e.g., rapid-fire pistol shooting, skeet and trap shooting, and the martial arts).

- Very low scores on negative affect expression (NAE), positive affect expression (PAE), self-esteem (SES), analytical ability (BIT), and need for control (CON) are associated with unrealistic expectations and an inability to own failure in a way that allows the person to change problem behavior. The ability to analyze equips the person with the ability to generate excuses and counterarguments to even constructive criticism. The high level of self-esteem and the need for control cause the person to trust his or her own judgment more than the judgment of others. As a result, the individual lacks the motivation to change, because he or she disagrees with analyses of others.

- High control (CON) combined with high self-esteem (SES) and balanced scores on the extroversion and introversion scales (EXT, INT) can create conflict for others. When Pete needs space and privacy, he will withdraw from involvement with others. If the people from whom he withdraws are emotionally dependent on him (e.g., his approval and involvement are important to them), they may take his withdrawal personally. Instead of recognizing that Pete needs personal space and privacy, they may feel he does not want to be around them.

Case 3—Water Polo Madness

Reason for Referral (Recap)

Howard is the talented water polo player who can't seem to control his anger in tight situations.

What is the athlete's most likely response set?
Because Howard was forced by the coach to come in, he may not have been the most cooperative person when filling out the inventory. However, his test scores are consistent with the problem described by the coach. In the interview, Howard should be asked about his attitude when taking the test. His motivation for change should also be investigated.

Does the athlete have the technical and tactical skill required to be successful?
The issue, as far as the coach is concerned, is clearly not a technical or tactical issue. Howard has the mental skills and knowledge; he is simply lacking the emotional control.

Interpretation Steps

What is the athlete's concentration strength and relative weakness?
Howard's concentration strength is his ability to see everything that is going on around him, then to react quickly and instinctively to changing conditions (BET). Howard's external awareness can be very helpful in a team sport like water polo, helping him find the open man or the opening he needs to take a shot. His relative weaknesses are his attention to detail and his follow-through (NAR). This suggests that Howard may have accomplished a great deal based on his talent rather than on hard work and self-discipline.

How confident, competitive, and willing to take control is the athlete?
Howard has a high need for control (CON) and is willing to take charge. He is very confident in his skills and abilities (SES) and highly competitive (P/O). Howard's competitive nature, confidence, and need for control, combined with his natural talent, have allowed him to achieve a high level of performance.

How quickly does the athlete make decisions?
Howard is a very quick decision maker (low OBS). This can help him in the pool when there isn't much time to think. When a situation requires a more thoughtful approach, however, Howard may be a bit too reactive (e.g., when running the clock out or while trying to preserve a one-goal lead).

Is the athlete extroverted, introverted, both, or neither?
Howard is "one of the boys." He is extroverted, outgoing, and likes to socialize. He enjoys being part of a team. You might use this fact to help him gain control over his anger.

How expressive is the athlete of thoughts, ideas, and feelings?
Howard holds nothing back. He is going to share his thoughts and feelings with you, whether you want to hear them or not (high IEX, NAE, PAE). He is so reactive to changes in his environment (BET) that one minute he behaves as if he loves you (PAE) and the next minute he seems to treat you like his worst enemy.

How easily does the athlete lose control over thoughts and feelings?
Howard's scores on the overload scales (OET, OIT, RED) are fairly low, which indicates that he does not see himself as losing control over his ability to concentrate. This is at odds with the loss of control over emotions that is getting him into trouble. Because Howard admits to expressing his feelings openly (NAE, PAE) and because he admits to "doing his own thing" (BCON), he doesn't perceive his expressions of anger and frustration as a loss of control. In his eyes, his anger and his behavior are justified.

Describe the athlete's strengths within the context of his performance environment.
Howard's high levels of control (CON), confidence (SES), and competitiveness (P/O), along with his willingness to challenge and confront others (NAE), make him a very aggressive and, at times, intimidating player. He does not give up easily. He'll fight to the end. When Howard has his emotions under control, he has an uncanny ability to see everything that is going on in the pool (BET). He has great instincts and can anticipate openings and the play of his opponents. Howard is extroverted and outgoing (EXT) and is capable of being supportive of other members of the team (PAE).

Describe the athlete's most likely performance error under increasing pressure.
Pressure increases for Howard when he starts to lose control over a situation or when he or the team doesn't play as well as he expects. When this happens, anger develops. Strong emotions narrow Howard's focus of attention. He loses any ability to think through the consequences of his actions before acting and even loses his sensitivity to everything around him except the

object of his anger (e.g., a particular opponent, an official, a teammate, himself).

What attentional and interpersonal factors contribute to the performance problem, and what steps can be taken by the athlete to improve?
Howard's need for control (CON), high self-confidence (SES), and high competitiveness (P/O) combine with his natural talent to set the stage for most of his problems. These are the same characteristics that drive him to be successful. When his need for control is threatened, or when he isn't receiving the recognition and respect he feels he deserves, he reacts emotionally.

Howard's emotions are intense (high NAE and PAE); he relies on intuition (BET, low OBS) rather than on taking time before he acts to think about the possible consequences of his behavior. Because his feelings of control and self-esteem remain high even when he loses emotional control, you should anticipate that working with him will not be easy. There are probably two reasons for this:

1. He undoubtedly feels that he should be able to solve all of his own problems, that he doesn't need help. If he can't do it, no one can.

2. He probably takes pride in his willingness to be open and honest with his thoughts and feelings. Whether he is happy or angry, he wants you to know it. There are times when it is so important to him that you know how he feels that nothing else matters, not even the outcome of the competition.

You will need to approach Howard by applauding his honesty and openness. You do not want to imply that you are asking him to change the way he sees himself (honest, with integrity) in order to gain greater control over his behavior. Any change should occur without Howard having to alter his perception of his honesty and openness. To succeed, you must help him find ways to keep the long-term consequences in sight. You must also persuade him to allow others to help him keep these consequences in mind. You may be able to do this by drawing on his need for involvement with others and his desire to be part of the team.

You should also be able to help Howard by getting him to realize that his anger is causing him to lose control over his greatest skill from a playing standpoint—his ability to see the entire pool. If you can enable Howard to recognize the negative impact his control issue has on qualities that are important to him, such as emotional honesty, you have a chance of effecting change.

What are the lessons to be learned from this case?
• There is a pattern of scores on TAIS associated with the impatience, frustration, and anger that cause many athletes to become their own worst enemy. Look for a high score on the competitiveness scale cluster (CON, SES, and P/O) and a low obsessive score/quick decision score (OBS). In addition, scores on the behavior control scale (BCON) and the negative affect expression scale (NAE) are elevated. A high BCON score means the individual has a tendency to behave in unconventional ways, to do things his or her own way. When you see this pattern, you can predict that for this individual, anger and frustration develop easily in the face of failure. The anger may be directed at an opponent, at officials, or at the athlete him-

or herself. The feelings become so strong that the athlete attacks, tries to get even, and often forgets about the importance of the outcome.

- When scores on the self-esteem scale (SES) and the control scale (CON) remain high in spite of an obvious problem, it is difficult to keep athletes motivated to change their behavior long enough to effect permanent change. Individuals with high control and self-esteem scores often believe they have control before they really do. These scores also make it difficult for them to accept outside help; this is especially true if the score on the self-critical scale (DEP) is very low.

- When the external awareness scale (BET) is the highest attentional scale, look at the other two attentional scales (BIT and NAR). The lower these scale scores, the more likely it is that the athlete is surviving on natural talent rather than on hard work and discipline (NAR) or on the ability to outthink (BIT) the opposition.

Case 4—Gymnastics Superstar

Reason for Referral (Recap)

Ludmilla is the Olympic champion and two-time world champion on the uneven parallel bars and is an odds-on favorite to repeat in the upcoming Olympics.

What is the athlete's most likely response set?
Given her experience and previous success, Ludmilla is unlikely to be defensive or to exaggerate strengths on the inventory. If she believes you have something to offer, she might exaggerate her weaknesses in order to help you identify areas in which she needs improvement.

Does the athlete have the technical and tactical skill required to be successful?
You do not need to be a coach or to understand much about the sport to recognize that an Olympic champion has the technical and tactical skill necessary to be successful. Her success has proven that already.

Interpretation Steps

What is the athlete's concentration strength and relative weakness?
Ludmilla's concentration strength is her ability to focus (NAR). For gymnastics, this is the skill that becomes most important. Ludmilla needs to practice her routine until it's perfect, until it can be executed automatically. Her low information processing score (INFP) indicates that she likes structure and prefers to focus on one thing at a time.

Ludmilla's analytical scale score (BIT) shows her relative weakness. Under pressure, Ludmilla may become too focused and inflexible. Her ability to problem-solve or to consider alternative approaches to a performance-related problem may suffer when she is stressed.

How confident, competitive, and willing to take control is the athlete?
Ludmilla scores high on the need-for-control scale (CON), but only average on the self-esteem scale (SES). The self-esteem score seems quite low for an Olympic and world champion. Clearly, Ludmilla is highly demanding and

critical of herself (average SES, relatively high DEP). Her competitiveness score is within the average range for world champions and suggests that she may have exaggerated what she perceives to be her weaknesses when she responded to TAIS.

How quickly does the athlete make decisions?
Ludmilla is a cautious decision maker (high OBS). She is a perfectionist and wants to avoid mistakes at all costs. Undoubtedly, her perfectionism and her focus (NAR) are two factors that have contributed significantly to her success.

Is the athlete extroverted, introverted, both, or neither?
Ludmilla is more introverted (INT) than extroverted (EXT). Her introversion has probably contributed both to her focus and to her willingness to work and train hard (fewer social distractions). It may also explain why her coach feels as though he doesn't really know her.

How expressive is the athlete of thoughts, ideas, and feelings?
Ludmilla does not express her thoughts and ideas (IEX), and she does not express anger (NAE). She will express positive feelings (PAE), but any anger she feels is kept inside and not shown to others (NAE). The coach may know how Ludmilla feels when she is happy and satisfied, but he is not likely to know how she feels when she is unhappy. (Given Ludmilla's perfectionism, she isn't going to be satisfied very often.)

How easily does the athlete lose control over thoughts and feelings?
Ludmilla has been hard on herself here. She has admitted a great deal of distractibility, from both external (OET) and internal (OIT) factors. She has also indicated that she has a tendency to become overly focused (RED), often failing to shift from an internal focus to an external one or vice versa.

The high score on RED combined with the high OBS score suggests that Ludmilla's concern about avoiding mistakes will seriously impair her performance when she has to make adjustments or "think on her feet." Fortunately, Ludmilla usually has time to settle herself down and to clear her thoughts before she begins her performance on the uneven parallel bars. She doesn't have to start her routine until she is ready. Once she starts, she goes on automatic pilot. Her performance will be affected in other areas (e.g., when she has to respond to questions by the press).

Describe the athlete's strengths within the context of her performance environment.
Ludmilla is extremely hardworking (NAR), dedicated (CON and P/O) perfectionist (OBS). She takes responsibility for her training (CON) and listens to others (average SES). Although highly demanding and critical of herself, she remains positive and supportive of others. She reacts to her own failure not with anger and frustration (low NAE) but with more focus and hard work (NAR).

Describe the athlete's most likely performance error under increasing pressure.
As pressure increases, Ludmilla communicates less and keeps her concerns to herself. On these occasions, she can become so narrowly focused that she is unable to step back and consider alternative ways of accomplishing

goals and objectives. She will grow stubborn and push herself harder and harder until her coach intervenes out of concern for her well-being.

What attentional and interpersonal factors contribute to the performance problem, and what steps can be taken by the athlete to improve?

Ludmilla's perfectionism (NAR, RED, OBS) is both her greatest strength (it has gotten her to the top) and her greatest weakness. Her perfectionism and drive make her susceptible to burnout because nothing will ever be good enough (SES, DEP). Her introverted nature (INT vs. EXT) keeps the pressure that she puts on herself inside (IEX, NAE, DEP, and SES) and prevents others from recognizing when she needs help or emotional support.

Ludmilla's relatively low self-confidence (SES), low analytical skill (BIT), and low intellectual expression (IEX) suggest that she is open to technical and tactical help from others. She undoubtedly trusts her coach's ability to problem-solve (e.g., to develop routines) more than she trusts her own.

In the interview, you will want to find out how much of Ludmilla's worry and obsessiveness (RED, OBS) is due to sport-related issues and how much is due to other, personal matters. She will undoubtedly trust her coach with the sport-related issues, but she may not be willing to share any personal problems. In order to help Ludmilla in both areas, you will need to find people she trusts and get them working together in a cooperative way by a) sensitizing them to the behavior Ludmilla displays when she is overly obsessive and focused and b) encouraging Ludmilla to take the risk of sharing some of her thoughts and feelings with them.

What are the lessons to be learned from this case?

- Perfectionism (NAR plus OBS), even when it is associated with a breakdown in the ability to shift concentration (RED), need not interfere with performance in a closed-skill sport, especially sports in which athletes have the luxury of waiting until they are ready to initiate performance. Sports like archery, golf, diving, gymnastics, bowling, and the jumps in track and field give the athlete a certain amount of freedom in terms of initiating an activity that once initiated, continues automatically. Often, elite-level performers in these sports have high scores on the RED scale; errors occur away from competition. For example, an athlete who is thinking about, obsessing over, or mentally practicing a routine when a parent, spouse, or teacher is giving directions is likely to make a mistake because critical information was missed.

- Introversion (INT), when combined with a high need for control (CON), a narrow focus of concentration (NAR), an obsession with perfectionism (OBS), and an intensely competitive nature (P/O), can lead to burnout and injury if left unchecked. Athletes with these qualities don't know when to relax and to take time out.

- The self-esteem scale (SES) is a good indicator of the openness of an individual to the input of others. The higher the level of self-esteem, the less confidence and trust the individual has in others' opinions and, hence, the less likely the athlete is to listen to opinions that contradict his or her own. The lower the level of self-esteem, the more the athlete trusts others and the less he or she trusts him- or herself. To interpret moderate self-esteem scores, look to other TAIS scales. In this case, the athlete lacks trust in her analytical skills (BIT) and in her ability to express her thoughts and ideas (IEX).

Case 5—Life on the Edge

Reason for Referral (Recap)

Heidi is the talented speed skier with a history of career-threatening injuries. Her coach has described her as extremely difficult to work with.

What is the athlete's most likely response set?
We would expect Heidi to cooperate with the assessment process. If she is as emotionally volatile as her coach says she is, we would expect her scores on TAIS to be somewhat more extreme and variable than those of most other athletes.

Does the athlete have the technical and tactical skill required to be successful?
Given the level at which she is skiing and the fact that the coach didn't identify any technical issues, we wouldn't anticipate any lack of skill.

Interpretation Steps

What is the athlete's concentration strength and relative weakness?
Heidi's concentration strength is her external awareness (BET), a skill that can be very important in speed skiing. She must be able to look down the course if she hopes to anticipate problems. Her relative weakness is her analytical skill (BIT). If her analytical score were any higher, she might never race, given the dangers associated with downhill skiing.

How confident, competitive, and willing to take control is the athlete?
Heidi is extremely confident (SES), competitive (P/O), and controlling (CON), even for a world-class athlete. Her need for control and her high level of self-confidence contribute to the difficulty the coach is facing in trying to work with her. She probably tries as hard to control and to set limits on him as he does with her.

How quickly does the athlete make decisions?
Heidi's speed of decision making is average (OBS). This, combined with her relatively high score on the focused attention scale (NAR), suggests that she is a very hard worker and that she prepares thoroughly for her races.

Is the athlete extroverted, introverted, both, or neither?
Heidi is much more extroverted than introverted; she needs to be around other people. Typically, athletes like Heidi—as extroverted as they are—can't help but constantly compete with others. They use the successes of others to motivate themselves to train harder. This can place a strain on friendships.

How expressive is the athlete of thoughts, ideas, and feelings?
Like most world-class athletes, Heidi is in the average range when it comes to expressing thoughts and ideas (IEX). When dealing with technical and tactical issues, she trusts her coach. Emotionally, however, she is explosive, with extremely high scores on both the positive affect expression scale (PAE) and the negative affect expression scale (NAE).

How easily does the athlete lose control over thoughts and feelings?
Although not easily distracted by environmental cues (OET), Heidi does get distracted by her own thoughts and feelings (OIT). Her high score on the behavior control scale (BCON), combined with her high score on negative affect expression (NAE), suggests that she can be quite emotionally explosive.

Describe the athlete's strengths within the context of her performance environment.
Heidi's external awareness (BET) and her attention to detail (NAR) serve her well as a speed skier. The relatively high score on the behavior control scale (BCON), combined with effective concentration skills, a high level of self-confidence, extreme competitiveness, and the belief that she is in control of situations, suggests that Heidi likes living on the edge, taking risks, and being different. Her reaction to pressure and to her own mistakes is likely to be anger; she undoubtedly uses this anger to get herself to ski faster.

Describe the athlete's most likely performance error under increasing pressure.
As pressure increases, Heidi throws caution to the wind. This is when she may not ski the best race tactically or technically, but she will probably ski fast. Her anger will take control, and if she doesn't injure herself, she may win the race. Off the slopes, her emotional expressiveness will create conflicts between her, her teammates, and the coaches. As major competitions get close, her emotions will take over, and she will make remarks that will hurt and anger others. Because of her high self-esteem, more often than not she will see the negative emotional reactions others have to what she says as being their problem: "They are too sensitive. They should understand where I am coming from."

What attentional and interpersonal factors contribute to the performance problem, and what steps can be taken by the athlete to improve?
The characteristics that make Heidi a great downhill skier are not the best characteristics for maintaining close friendships and relationships. Heidi is very sensitive and reactive to the environment. She is a highly competitive, highly emotional individual who has achieved success by using her anger to push herself beyond the limits most people set for themselves. For Heidi, there is no compromising, especially under pressure. Either she is totally involved and committed, or she is not there at all. When she is totally involved, she is extremely demanding of herself and of others.

We have serious questions about suggesting changes to Heidi, at least as long as she wants to compete. For Heidi to change, she would have to take more time to think about the consequences of her actions, both for herself and for others. Encouraging her to think more seriously about such things, and getting her to care more about the feelings of others, would probably make her more vulnerable and cautious as a skier.

If Heidi had a significant technical or tactical advantage over the other skiers, she could ski more conservatively and still win. Without that technical or tactical advantage, however, winning boils down to who is willing to push him- or herself just a little closer to the absolute limit.

From a relationship standpoint, the best way to help Heidi and her coach is to provide both of them with a better understanding of how her behavior affects her skiing, then to emphasize to both of them that quality communication will take place only under relatively nonstressful conditions.

In the interview, you will want to find out if winning, to Heidi, is worth the risk of injuries. If it is, then the most you can do in terms of controlling her anger is to try to ensure that it is appropriately directed when she steps into the starting gate.

What are the lessons to be learned from this case?

- Anger, in and of itself, is not a bad thing. Some athletes, like Heidi, are able to use it quite effectively to help themselves perform. Taking away their anger can be like taking away their engine.

- It is common to see a fairly high score on the behavior control scale (BCON) and on negative affect expression (NAE) with athletes who are involved in high-risk sports. In addition, many of these athletes are easily distracted, both externally (OET) and internally (OIT)—some even more than Heidi. It is as if they need a high-risk environment to be able to concentrate. Distractibility is reduced during competition, because competition raises the adrenaline levels enough to allow such athletes to focus. When this happens, they will usually have high control and self-esteem scores (CON and SES) in spite of high scores on the overload scores. If an individual is distractible and both self-esteem and control are low, this interpretation does not hold, and chances are that the athlete is not succeeding.

Case 6—The Moody Striker

Reason for Referral (Recap)

Sarah is the talented striker on her college soccer team who was voted league MVP for the past 2 years. She has noticed that just prior to the onset of menstruation, she has difficulty concentrating and feels less energetic than at other times.

What is the athlete's most likely response set?
Because she is self-referred, Sarah would have worked hard to identify the items in the inventory that would help to differentiate her feelings at the two different times of the month. If the inventory measures performance-relevant characteristics as it is supposed to, the differences between the two test occurrences should provide a clear picture of what is happening psychologically with Sarah just prior to menstruation.

Does the athlete have the technical and tactical skill required to be successful?
Yes.

Interpretation Steps

What is the athlete's concentration strength and relative weakness (midcycle vs. premenstrual)?
Sarah has exceptional concentration skills midcycle, her strength being her ability to focus her concentration (NAR). Her relative weakness would be her

external awareness, but this is still at the 80th percentile. The major change from midcycle to premenstrual is a dramatic increase in Sarah's external distractibility (OET) and a corresponding decrease in her ability to narrow her concentration (NAR). Sarah's strength just prior to menstruation is her ability to analyze (BIT), which is only slightly negatively affected by her menstrual cycle and which drops from 93% midcycle to 83%.

How confident, competitive, and willing to take control is the athlete (midcycle vs. premenstrual)?
Midcycle, Sarah feels in control (CON=85%), extremely confident (SES=99%), and very competitive (P/O=95%). Just prior to menstruation, Sarah feels less competitive (60%) and very much out of control (22%).

How quickly does the athlete make decisions (midcycle vs. premenstrual)?
Sarah's speed of decision making, which falls within the average range both for the general population and for athletes involved in open-skill sports, is unaffected by her menstrual cycle.

Is the athlete extroverted, introverted, both, or neither (midcycle vs. premenstrual)?
Sarah is more of an extrovert (EXT=70%) than an introvert (INT=22%). This remains true just prior to menstruation; however, her score on the extroversion scale does drop to 50%.

How expressive is the athlete of thoughts, ideas, and feelings (midcycle vs. premenstrual)?
Midcycle, Sarah is highly verbal (95%). This score drops dramatically just prior to menstruation (to 50%). For most of the month, Sarah is significantly more positive in her emotional expression (PAE=73% vs. NAE=32%). Just prior to menstruation, there is a decrease in her expression of positive feelings and an increase in negative ones (PAE=55%, NAE=55%). Finally, Sarah's self-critical score shifts from the 12th percentile (not very self-critical) to the 78th percentile just prior to menstruation.

How easily does the athlete lose control over thoughts and feelings (midcycle vs. premenstrual)?
Looking at Sarah's scores on the attentional scales and on BCON and NAE, she appears to lose more control premenstrually over her ability to focus and shift concentration than over her expression of emotions (though both are affected). Premenstrually, Sarah is significantly more distractible, less positive, and more negative. This loss of control is reflected directly in her score on the control scale, which drops from 85% midcycle to 22% premenstrual.

Describe the athlete's strengths within the context of her performance environment (midcycle only).
Sarah is an exceptional competitor (P/O) and someone who won't give up (SES). She works extremely hard to develop her skills (NAR). She can be very strategic in her thinking on the field (BIT) and has exceptional external awareness as well (BET). Her moderately high control score (CON) indicates she can follow as well as lead. Outgoing and positive (EXT, PAE), she fits in well with the other members of the team. She expects a lot of herself and is a positive role model for others.

Describe the athlete's most likely performance error under increasing pressure (premenstrual only).

Just prior to menstruation, Sarah is more likely to make mistakes because she loses some awareness of performance-relevant external cues (BET) and because she gets distracted by things going on around her (OET) and by her own thoughts and feelings. At such times, she is less likely to assert herself and take a leadership role (CON, P/O) and may present a more cautious, negative image to her teammates.

What attentional and interpersonal factors contribute to the performance problem, and what steps can be taken by the athlete to improve?

Based on her scores, just prior to menstruation Sarah begins to have trouble separating signal (task-relevant cues, BET) from noise (OET, OIT). The drop in her score on the information-processing scale (INFP goes from 95% down to 80%) suggests that she has less energy and is less capable of coping with several things at once. Sarah's feelings of being out of control (CON) are probably exaggerated (i.e., others would not see the decrease in her ability to perform that she feels). The most obvious signal to others that Sarah is experiencing problems would probably be her decreased expressiveness (IEX) and the change in her attitude—less positive and more negative.

Before attempting to change anything, you must determine the extent to which Sarah's play is significantly affected, both in her eyes and in the eyes of others. Because Sarah is so analytical and is always looking for ways to improve, you need to find out what steps she has already taken to try to control the changes that occur in her ability to concentrate and in her feelings just prior to menstruation. If the changes are hormonal or biochemical, you probably will not have much success with psychological interventions. You may, however, be able to provide some relief by reducing the expectations that Sarah and others place on her at the difficult time in her cycle. You can do this by helping her to adjust her priorities so that they are consistent with the changes in her ability to process information and to multitask.

What are the lessons to be learned from this case?

- Do not underestimate the ability of an individual to use an inventory like TAIS to contrast his or her ability to process information and communicate with others under different conditions or situations. Information gained this way can be very useful in enhancing the respondent's self-awareness and in improving communication between the respondent and significant others.

Suggested Readings

Evans, I. (1993). Constructional perspectives in clinical assessment. *Psychological Assessment, 5,* 264–272.

Nideffer, R. M. (1993). *The Attentional & Interpersonal Style Inventory (TAIS): Theory and application.* New Berlin, WI: ASI Publications.

Nideffer, R. M. (1993). Concentration and attention control training. In J. Williams (Ed.), *Applied sport psychology* (pp. 243–262). Mountain View, CA: Mayfield.

Pratt, R. W., & Nideffer, R. M. (1993). *Taking care of business.* New Berlin, WI: Assessment Systems International.

Developing Your Interviewing and Test Feedback Skills

7

The ability to consensually validate test results and to provide feedback in a useful and compelling way is more art than science. In this chapter, we will provide you with a structure you can use in a feedback session to

- validate and refine your interpretations of TAIS scores,

- assess the individual's level of motivation to change,

- determine the likelihood that the individual will be able to change, and

- make recommendations and begin to develop a performance-improvement program.

We will also explain how to use role-playing to develop the intuitive and artistic side of the feedback process. How far you progress in this area will depend on the amount of practice you are willing to engage in. In addition to having performance-relevant information to give to the client, you need to have your own act together psychologically. Here are some of the psychological skills that differentiate feedback artists from feedback technicians:

- Artists are able to "park their egos" outside the interview room.

- Artists are aware of, and able to "put on" (mirror), the nonverbal behaviors of their clients.

- Artists are confident in their ability to control the emotional arousal and defensiveness of the client.

- Artists confront issues head-on and are able to do so in terms the athlete can relate to and understand.

Parking Your Ego

Nothing will interfere more with your ability to control what goes on in a feedback session than concern about your own performance. The feedback session isn't about you; it's about and for the person to whom you are providing the feedback. The more you worry about your own performance, the less capable you are of making good behavioral observations and of really hearing what the other person is telling you. If you think about it, this is just an extension of the relationship we talked about between level of arousal, focus of concentration, and performance. Anxiety about your performance causes you to develop a narrow internal focus of concentration; as a result, you lose some of your ability to attend to the client.

It's easy to tell you to forget about your own issues and to focus totally on the client, but how do you do that? You probably won't be able to do it right away. The ability to control anxiety and set your own issues aside is itself a skill that must be developed. It is the same skill your clients must master to improve their performance. Here are four steps that will help you gain confidence and control in feedback sessions:

1. **Simplify your role.** Do this by providing yourself with a simple structure that guides you through the feedback session, a structure that doesn't require much complex problem-solving and analysis on your part. You need to know what you want to cover in the session and how you want to cover it. We will provide you with that structure. Once you are comfortable doing it our way, you'll have something to fall back on if you become anxious; as a result, you'll feel more comfortable making changes, going off in your own direction, and improvising.

2. **Develop simple skills to avoid distractions, to reduce your level of arousal, and to refocus your attention on the task at hand.** We use simple breathing techniques and the process of centering to reduce arousal and to redirect focus of concentration. (For additional information on centering, see Nideffer, 1992.)

3. **Have some ready-made excuses you can use to literally take time out during the feedback session.** Even the best performers have times when they lose it. Sometimes they just aren't ready to perform. If they try to force the performance, they fail. Athletes learn to find excuses they can use to delay things long enough for them to pull themselves together. They suddenly have to tie a shoelace, or they get a cramp that magically goes away. They have to go to the bathroom, they lose their mouthpiece in a fight, or they clinch and hold on. As an interviewer, you need to have several delaying strategies available. You may never have to use them, but just knowing they are there can provide enough comfort to settle you down and allow you to continue.

4. **Practice, practice, practice.** There is no substitute for experience. Do not limit your practice to actual feedback situations or to role-playing. If you really want to improve, become a better observer of other people's interactions. Watch them. Try to be aware of what they are feeling as they talk. Notice how sensitive or insensitive they are to each other. What cues are they reading? Can you predict what direction the conversation will take? Can you see ways to improve their communication process? Can you plot their TAIS profiles or their profiles on the other tests you use, based on your observations?

Developing Sensitivity to Client Nonverbal Behavior

Being an artist requires a sixth sense for what the client is thinking and feeling. In most situations, you will want to be more concerned with how a client says something than with what the client says. It's how things are said that enables you to determine an athlete's ability to cope with pressure and to gauge his or her level of motivation and ability to change behavior.

Built into your brain are stimulus patterns that are associated with different emotional expressions, expressions you have learned to interpret. When we talk about "putting on," or mirroring, the nonverbal behavior of a person, we are telling you to observe your client's behavior and then to assume a similar posture, facial expression, rate of breathing, level of muscle tension, and tone of voice. Then ask yourself what you feel. Once you know what the person is feeling, examine the situational context to determine what could have triggered these feelings.

You need not limit your practice of this technique to feedback interviews. You can observe people in the "real world" (e.g., at another table in a restaurant) and practice. If you do, you will find that before long you won't have to actually identify with the other person's position to know what he or she is feeling. Mentally, you can trigger the stimulus pattern just by observing what is happening.

Controlling the Client's Level of Emotional Arousal

You will want to learn how much pressure it takes before the athlete loses control over dominant concentration skills and intra- and interpersonal characteristics. If you can determine this, and you know the concentration skills and interpersonal characteristics required by the athlete's sport, then you can predict the conditions under which that individual will and will not perform well.

Not only is it necessary for you to know how much pressure it takes before an athlete begins to lose control, but you also want to get an idea of how difficult it is for the athlete to regain control once he or she has started to lose it. You can begin to answer both of these questions by manipulating the amount of pressure the athlete feels during your feedback interview, and then by observing the resultant behavior.

Athletes react to increasing pressure in one of two ways. Those who are highly confident react with frustration or anger. Those who lack confidence react with anxiety or self-doubt. For many people, the thought of making someone else anxious or angry is itself anxiety-producing. Most people want to get along, so they try to avoid making others uncomfortable. The fact is, if you are going to be helpful, you will sometimes have to make people uncomfortable. All people become uncomfortable when confronted with failure; with the unexpected or unknown; or with challenges to their integrity, intelligence, or honesty.

If you can learn to mirror the feelings of the athletes you work with, you will be able to sense to what degree you can, and should, confront them. You'll also learn how you can use your nonverbal and verbal behavior to increase or decrease the amount of pressure you put on the athlete. Remember to always keep this type of manipulation within reason, so you can maintain an effective working relationship.

Using TAIS Results to Predict Behavior in the Feedback Session

One of the exercises we will ask you to perform in this chapter is to look at an athlete's TAIS profile, then use the profile to try to anticipate how the athlete will behave in the feedback session. To do this, you "put on the pro-file." You imagine yourself with the same concentration skills, the same level of confidence, the same need for control, the same speed of decision making, and the same level of expressiveness as the athlete's. Given these characteristics, you ask yourself how you would behave if challenged during the feedback session. Would you react with anger, or would you become anxious? What effect would the challenge have on your posture, your facial expression, your tone of voice, and your expressiveness?

The more skilled you become at anticipating the athlete's behavior in the interview, the more control you'll have over the interview. Just as you can anticipate how the individual will respond to a challenge, so can you anticipate how he or she will respond to support.

Assessing the Athlete's Level of Emotional Control

You don't need to push people to the point of losing control to get a sense of how easily they can become upset or to determine how quickly and easily they recover from a threat, a mistake, or an emotional upset. There will be times during feedback when you will need to question the athlete's ability to perform under certain conditions. You will have to probe to find where the weaknesses are. Although he or she may want to improve, if the athlete is like most people, he or she still won't be happy when his or her abilities are questioned. As you address possible issues, ask yourself following questions to improve your observation skills:

- How quickly do emotions develop (e.g., anger or anxiety) when you question the athlete's abilities? What nonverbal cues signal these emotions in the athlete?

- How much defensiveness and denial does the athlete engage in? What excuses does he or she make for the behavior? Does the athlete merely disagree? Is the behavior consistent with the athlete's test scores?

- If you are skeptical about an answer the athlete gives you, and you show it in any of the following ways, how does the athlete react and how intense do his or her emotions become?

  - Telling the individual straight out that you don't believe what he or she is saying.

  - Rolling your eyes and muttering something like "Right."

  - Shaking your head and lifting your eyebrows, while saying something like "Really, you're a better person than I am. I wouldn't be able to do that. How do you manage?"

- Be careful to observe how quickly the athlete's anger or anxiety is reduced when you provide structure and support. How easy is it to redirect the athlete's attention, to get him or her to let go of the anxiety or anger by empathizing, agreeing, and then redirecting focus to another topic or to another way of looking at the issue?

Once the session is over, analyze your reactions to the athlete. How easy was it to begin to generate an emotion like anger or anxiety? How did any emotional changes affect the athlete's ability to analyze, to make decisions, to problem-solve, or to communicate with you? Will the athlete face similar or more difficult challenges in competitive situations? What would be the consequences of a loss of control in a competitive situation? How much did the athlete depend on you for help in regaining control of his or her emotions? Will or can the athlete develop the support he or she needs in the competitive environment to regain control, if control is lost? How can you help with that?

Remember, you are not trying to get the athlete to lose control; you are, however, trying to get a clear sense of how much pressure it takes to cause this to happen. If you have pushed as hard as you think the athlete is pushed during competition, and the athlete has managed to maintain control, there is no need to push harder. If you have been very gentle in your challenge but the athlete has reacted strongly, you don't need to push further, because you have attained the information you need.

Confronting Possible Issues

Skilled service providers are able to confront difficult issues with their clients in a way that minimizes defensiveness and maximizes the likelihood that something positive will result from the discussion. To help you develop this skill, we will provide you with eight steps (see Table 6, p. 128) to follow as you explore possible issues and attempt to encourage athletes to face issues. We have organized your interpretation of TAIS data (from the previous chapter) so that the analysis prepares you for this eight-step process.

Structuring the Feedback Interview

Before we take you through each of the steps outlined in Table 6, we would like to make some suggestions about structuring your feedback sessions with clients. There are many ways to provide feedback. The structure we suggest has been useful to us, and we believe it's a good place to start. Once you are comfortable with the assessment tools you are using and feel comfortable and in control in feedback sessions, you can develop your own method.

Session Length

If you are merely providing feedback and attempting to consensually validate results, 1 hour should be enough. If you are also developing a performance-improvement program, allow at least another hour.

Providing Test Information

If you have done a good job of interpreting the inventory and identifying key issues, there is no need to give the individual any test materials; in fact, handing a client a test profile can be distracting and time consuming. You'll end up having to explain each scale, how to read the profile, etc. All of this detracts from the focus you want the client to have on the critical issues at hand.

We usually provide our clients with a description of the issue and what contributes to it, without using any TAIS scale abbreviations. We also provide our recommendation, in writing. If a client is particularly interested in the psychology of sport and is keen on learning more, we may provide one of our TAIS computer-generated reports; we only do this, however, if we are convinced that doing so will not overload the athlete with information.

There are times when we provide a more formal report; for example, we may be asked to prepare a report for use as part of a selection process. At times, we encounter clinical issues that we need to refer to others. On these occasions, we write a report. That report is written to a third party, either to another professional (e.g., clinician, marriage-and-family counselor) or to someone we have trained—someone who we know will put what we say in the report into an appropriate perspective and who is well aware of the need to consensually validate our impressions. In chapter 9, we provide some guidelines for writing reports to third parties.

Physical Positioning

It is important for you to treat the athlete with respect and to expect the athlete to treat you the same way. You are equals, but with different areas of expertise. In our practice, we sit as equals; we don't sit behind a desk or in a bigger chair than the athlete does. If we are all sitting at a table, we either sit beside the athlete or across the table from him or her. We do not sit at the head of the table.

Taking Notes

We find having a notepad helpful. First, we can use note taking, or the illusion of note taking, as one of those time-out techniques we suggested you use when you need a break to pull your thoughts together. Second, we like to jot down our reactions to what the athlete says and does in the interview. We do this because our own emotional reactions can tell us a great deal about the way the athlete is seen by others.

To try to analyze our feelings during the interview would distract us from attending to the athlete. By taking notes during the session, we can recall key points and then analyze them. For example, if an athlete's reaction to something we say in the interview causes us to feel defensive, we need to figure out why. The interview, however, is not the time for us to do that. During the interview, we'll have to quickly let go of any defensiveness, accept what the athlete says, and move on. After the interview, we must determine whether the defensiveness we felt was justified on the basis of the athlete's behavior, or if we were simply being too sensitive. In other words, is it the athlete's problem or is it ours?

If we plan to work with the athlete in the future, we take notes so we can follow up on promises we make, and so we can make sure the athlete follows up on promises he or she makes. Having the notepad there also allows us to write items down for the athlete, to ensure that he or she understands and follows through on our recommendations and performance-enhancement plan.

Finally, we like having a notepad in front of us when we confront potential problem areas because it is one of the tools we can use to subtly increase and decrease the pressure the athlete is feeling. For example, if we express disagreement with a statement an athlete makes (e.g., "Are you sure? I find that hard to believe. I know I wouldn't interpret the coach's behavior that way.") and, at the same time, write something on our notepad, this raises the athlete's level of arousal. On the other hand, if we agree strongly with something the athlete says and write that down, our note-taking lowers the level of arousal. If we want to write something, but we do not want the athlete to make the connection between what we are writing and what is going on at that moment, we wait until a more comfortable or neutral time to record our thoughts.

The bottom line is, take notes! Just make sure that taking notes does not interfere with your ability to make good behavioral observations or to establish a relationship with the athlete.

Beginning the Feedback Session

If you haven't already established a relationship with the athlete, you'll want to take a few minutes to do this (or to start this process). If the athlete doesn't know much about us, we provide just enough information to give him or her a reason to place some confidence in what we have to say. That's usually not more than three or four sentences. What happens next depends on (a) how the individual came to us (i.e., did the individual seek us out on his or her own, or did someone else tell the individual to come to us?) and (b) whether there is a presenting problem unique to the individual.

Self-Referral With a Specific Problem

- If we have not already received a thorough description of the problem from the athlete, we'll ask him or her to tell us about it: *"You mentioned over the phone that you were concerned about _____ . Can you tell us more about your concerns?"*

- We want the athlete to provide information about his or her sport and about where and when problems occur. This will allow us to direct test feedback to specific examples to which the athlete can relate. As soon as we feel we have enough information to allow us to connect TAIS findings to actual behavior, we'll begin the feedback process by saying something like *"That's helpful. Let us tell you what we've inferred from your responses to the inventory we asked you to fill out."*

- If we already have a fairly thorough description of the problem, we'll summarize what we have discussed as being the issue and check with the client to make sure that our summary is accurate. If we understand the problem well enough, we should already have enough specific performance examples to connect to the results from testing: *"Good, all right, let us tell you what we've gotten from your responses to the inventory we asked you to fill out."*

Self-Referral With No Specific Problem

- There are times when people self-refer simply because they know psychological factors are important and think we have information that will be helpful. Even when this seems like a plausible reason, we'll often start with a bit of a challenge: *"The fact that you are coming to see us says that you aren't 100% satisfied with your performance. Where do you think you can improve?"* We'll also ask a general question about the sport to get information about potential problem areas, the kind of concentration skills required, etc.: *"Tell us a little about your sport. What do you think are the differences between really great players in your sport and those who are just good?"*

- Once we have gathered enough information about the sport to know the kind of problems that develop and the circumstances under which they develop, we are in a position to begin providing test feedback: *"Okay, let us tell you what we've learned about you from your responses to the inventory."*

Other Referral With a Specific, Individual Problem

- When an athlete does not self-refer, it's important for us to spend a little extra time establishing a relationship. It's also important for us to establish trust as quickly as possible. We will pave the way for doing that by first asking the person making the referral how much that person is sharing with us and what he or she has already shared with the athlete. If the referring person has not shared anything, we will ask the individual to share as much as he or she is comfortable with; we will then request permission to relay to the athlete what that person has told us.

- Our goal when we meet with the athlete is to be able to say something like the following: *"What has coach ____ told you about the reasons she wanted you to come and see us?"* We'll listen to the athlete's response, and then we'll say something like *"That's close to our understanding"* or *"That's not exactly how it was explained to us."* In either case, our next line is *"Let us tell you everything we know. We encourage you to jump in and ask questions or present another point of view whenever you feel like it."*

- As the process continues, we gain knowledge about the sport, about the kinds of problems that develop, and about the situations that lead to those problems. If the athlete agrees with the coach on the issue, we will begin providing TAIS feedback, tying it to the problem and to possible solutions.

- If the athlete denies problems, but TAIS information and the athlete's interview behavior suggest that problems exist, we'll begin TAIS feedback. Our goal during the feedback process will be to get the athlete to begin to see what others are seeing.

- If the athlete denies problems, and TAIS information and the athlete's behavior with us suggest that the problems lie with the person making the referral rather than with the athlete, we have a dilemma. We must take time out to come up with a way either to end the session or to approach the real issue without doing further damage to the relationship between the referring person and the athlete.

Other Referral With No Specific, Individual Problem

- This situation usually occurs when a coach—or an organization—has a strong belief that an entire team could be performing better, and the referring source wants some help. For example, the coach of a professional baseball team asked us to work with his hitters because he knew that concentration was important and could always be improved. In a sense, there was a reason for referral, but it was not specific to an individual, and we didn't know if the individuals being referred would accept our help.

- There should always be a reason for testing and a reason for working with an athlete. In this situation, we need to ask the athletes how enthusiastic they are about seeing us: *"Coach asked us to test and meet with all of the members of the team because he felt the information we could provide would help everyone improve concentration skills and their ability to communicate and support one another. How do you feel about that? Do you think we can help you or any of the others on the team?"*

- Let's say the athlete says, "No, I don't need any help." We'll then challenge that statement in order to learn a little more about the sport and about pressure situations in the sport: *"Really? You mean there's never been a situation where you haven't performed up to the level you're capable of? We've worked with the best athletes in the world, and none of them has ever said that to us. How do you manage to stay on top of everything all the time?"*

- If the athlete continues to resist, and we think we know enough about his or her sport to tie some of the TAIS findings to specific performance situations, we'll begin providing feedback. We'll introduce it in a challenging way, however: *"Well, as long as we're here, let us give you some feedback based on the inventory you took. Your scores did indicate that you have some real strengths, but there do appear to be some areas where you could improve."*

Eight Steps for Providing Test Feedback

Once we are past the introductions and we have gathered enough information from the athlete to provide us with sport-specific examples of the types of performance errors that occur within the sport and the conditions under which they occur, we'll begin the feedback process. We must accomplish several tasks during the session in order to be helpful. We must

- define the problem,

- communicate a clear understanding of the problem to the athlete,

- determine the athlete's willingness and ability to do something about the problem, and

- provide specific steps the athlete can take to address and to overcome the problem.

If you follow the eight steps outlined in Table 6, you will be able to accomplish these goals.

1. Describe *the individual's concentration abilities and intra- and interpersonal strengths.*
Most athletes, even those who want feedback for improvement, have a tendency to become defensive when someone challenges their ability to

Table 6. Eight Steps for Probing Possible Issues and Confronting Problem Areas

Describe	the individual's concentration abilities and intra- and interpersonal strengths.
Educate	the individual about what happens as pressure increases, how people lose flexibility and begin to rely too heavily on their dominant concentration and intra- and interpersonal skills.
Empathize	with the problems the individual is having by "owning" them yourself and by attributing them to others you have worked with (with similar test scores).
Probe	to see how accurate your sense of an existing or potential problem is by asking direct questions.
Validate	the individual's responses both verbally and nonverbally. Are they consistent with predictions made from TAIS scores?
Assess	the extent to which the individual is willing and able to make needed changes in behavior.
Identify	the steps the individual has already taken to cope with the problem(s).
Recommend	specific steps the individual can take to gain greater control over behavior.

perform. When people become defensive, their focus of attention turns inward. They begin to create a defense or prepare to go on the attack; in either case, they stop listening to what is being said. You can't communicate effectively with people if you can't get them to listen. To maximize the likelihood that individuals will listen to anything critical that you have to say and will be able to put it into a proper perspective, be sure they are relatively relaxed before you challenge them.

You begin to relax a person by establishing a relationship, by getting the athlete to tell you a little about his or her sport, and then by providing him or her with positive feedback from the inventory. If an athlete has been anxious about what the inventory might reveal, some positive feedback up front helps to reduce that anxiety. Positive feedback, when provided within the context of the athlete's sport and tied to some of the performance behaviors the athlete has described to you, helps to increase the athlete's confidence in you and in the inventory. We will illustrate this step, and the others, once we have defined them all.

2. Educate *the individual about what happens as pressure increases.*
Nothing makes an athlete more defensive than the feeling of being singled out or personally attacked. By taking a little time to let the athlete know that as pressure increases, everyone has a tendency to rely on highly developed skills and characteristics, you can reduce the likelihood that the athlete will take what follows as a personal attack.

As you will see when we go through the education process with John (Case 1), it is important for you to communicate the following points:

- Athletes are taught to practice physical skills until they are "overlearned." The reason they practice so long and so hard is that once a skill becomes automatic, it is much less likely to break down under increasing pressure—the athlete can still perform the skill when the heat is on.

- Concentration skills and interpersonal behaviors are learned, just like physical skills. The ones that have been practiced the most are the last ones to break down under pressure. Unfortunately, the strongest concentration skills and interpersonal characteristics are not always the ones most appropriate during competition.

- As concentration begins to break down under pressure, three error patterns occur:
    1. Rushing errors—
       The athlete consistently makes mistakes because he or she reacts too quickly or too intensely.
    2. Tentative errors—
       The athlete consistently makes mistakes because he or she fails to react or reacts with insufficient intensity.
    3. A combination of the two—
       Some athletes bounce back and forth, trying too hard one minute and failing to react quickly enough the next. The type of mistake an athlete is most likely to make is predictable based on TAIS scores.

The information you provide here can be invaluable to the athlete and can really add to your credibility. You should be able to describe each of the errors in terms the athlete can relate to and tie them directly to mistakes the athlete has either made him- or herself (according to the athlete) or has seen others in his or her sport make. For example, if your client is a diver, you might say,

> Watch a diver who is anxious and has some doubts about her ability to get all the way around when throwing a 2½. Chances are the anxiety and doubt will cause her to rush. Her anxiety will cause her to feel as if things are speeded up. She'll move faster on her approach, almost running to the end of the board. As she goes up in the air on her hurdle step, she'll be thinking about how hard she has to throw the dive to get around. As a result, she'll have problems waiting for the diving board to give her the lift she needs. She'll be trying to spring back up into the air while the board is still going down. That will keep her from getting the lift she needs. To make matters worse, increasing neck and shoulder muscle tension will keep her from getting the rotation she needs."

3. Empathize *with the individual by "owning" problems yourself or, better, by attributing them to others you have worked with or observed who are world-class performers in the same sport. Do not do this in a way that betrays confidentiality.*

As you begin to describe a problem you believe the athlete is likely to have, based on TAIS scores, do it by painting a picture. This picture should allow the athlete to see the inappropriate behavior as a natural consequence, something to be expected under the circumstances, not something to be ashamed of. The challenge for the athlete (and for you, now) is to develop the skill necessary to prevent that natural consequence from occurring, because natural or not, it is interfering with performance.

Paint your picture by taking the information you prepared prior to the session (when you identified the attentional and interpersonal factors that contribute to performance problems for the individual) and tying it directly to sport-specific performance issues the athlete has identified. Remember to use yourself or others in your example. Knowing that others have similar problems and reactions makes it easier for an athlete to accept his or her own; this is especially true if those others are people the athlete respects and admires. Telling an aspiring young athlete that someone he or she admires has had similar problems (without betraying any confidentiality) reduces defensiveness. When an athlete learns that the person you are referring to is also working on the issue, motivation usually increases. You can use yourself as an example, but make sure you do it in a way that is acceptable to the athlete. For example, if we tried to convince a world-record holder in diving that we had experienced similar things when we were diving, we would probably lose, rather than gain, credibility. Our level of diving would be so far below hers that it would be a joke. If, however, we can relate her problem to our performance experiences in a compelling way, she will be more apt to listen. For example,

> Susan, never having been there, I can only guess at the feelings you have when you're up on the tower. I have, however, been in other high-pressure situations, and I know there are some changes that take place in both concentration and physiology that are common across sports and across performance situations. Let me describe those in a sport I am familiar with and show you how they affect performance. Then you can see if they fit for your sport.

4. Probe *to see how accurate your sense of an existing or potential problem is by asking direct questions.*
This is a critical phase of the feedback process, and it is here that you will

- gather the information you need to validate your predictions,

- assess the athlete's level of motivation to make the kind of changes you feel he or she needs to make, and

- identify any steps the athlete has already taken to try to control the problem.

  Here are some of the questions we ask:

- *Does the picture we have just painted describe the kind of mistakes you find yourself making?*

- *If so, can you give us a couple of recent examples where this problem occurred? Is there any pattern to the problem, any situation where it is more likely to occur?*

- *If not, help us understand why not. Your scores on TAIS indicate ___. It's been our experience that this type of problem happens with some reg-*

ularity with other athletes who score as you have. Any idea as to why you are different?

If the athlete denies the existence of a problem, it's time to turn up the pressure to see if you can get the behavior to begin to emerge in the interview itself. Questioning the athlete's denial will increase his or her level of arousal. The more openly skeptical you are, the more that arousal will increase.

5. Validate *the individual's responses both verbally and nonverbally.*
If TAIS scores indicate that the athlete will deny weakness and will become frustrated or angry if you challenge the denial, look for evidence of this in the probing phase of the feedback session. If TAIS scores predict the athlete will have difficulty taking the initiative to express thoughts and feelings in the interview, is this what you find? Do you feel as if you have to pull everything out of the athlete? You predict that under pressure the athlete will respond to questions with simple answers and will agree with almost anything you say; is this the behavior you see in the feedback session? Do the behaviors you see in the interview occur on the playing field? If so, how would you recognize them? What specific behaviors would you see? Does the athlete "own" (acknowledge) that behavior out on the playing field? Can the individual provide you with specific examples of the kind of problems this behavior has created for him or her? By listening and watching, you will quickly attain a sense for whether or not your predictions and initial hypotheses have merit.

6. Assess *the extent to which the athlete is willing and able to make needed changes in behavior.*
If you are convinced that a problem exists, but the athlete refuses to see it, there is very little hope for change. About the only way to control the behavior is to keep the athlete out of situations in which it is a problem. If you are convinced that a problem exists, and the athlete agrees, then you are halfway there. Now you must ascertain whether the athlete believes the problem is serious enough to work on and whether the athlete believes he or she has the ability to overcome it. You might ask the following questions of the athlete:

- *Is the problem worth working on?*

- *How long has the problem existed?*

- *When mistakes occur, how obvious are they to you and to others?*

- *How long does it take you to regain control once you start making mistakes?*

- *What opportunity is there to get others involved in providing support and working with you to help you make gain greater control over your behavior?*

The answers to these questions will provide insight into how difficult it will be for the athlete to change. As you assess an individual's ability to change, keep the following in mind:

- The easiest way to correct poor performance is to avoid the performance situation. Is avoidance of the situation possible? It may be, if the individual is involved in a team sport and you can make a substitution or change his or her position.

- Most problems result from interactions between the individual and others. When this is the case, you need support from the environment to help the athlete make needed changes. Are such environmental supports available? Are there people who will help the athlete recognize when his or her behavior is getting out of control? Who will recognize changes the athlete is trying to make, encourage those changes, and reinforce the athlete for making them?

- Getting an athlete to change a long-established behavior pattern is a difficult task. Remember that you are not trying to eliminate a behavior. You would not want to eliminate thinking just because an athlete has a tendency to think too much under pressure. You only want to ensure that the behavior doesn't occur at an inappropriate time. The more predictable a problem is (e.g., because it always occurs under the same conditions), the easier it will be for the athlete to gain control.

- The easier it is for you to elicit problem behavior during the feedback session and the harder you must work to help the athlete move away from that behavior pattern once it develops, the poorer the prognosis for change.

7. Identify the steps the individual has already taken to cope with the problem(s).

Ask what the athlete has tried to do to gain control over an identified problem. The steps an athlete has already tried and their impact on the problem, or lack of it, will tell you a great deal. If he or she has tried a strategy you feel should work, and it hasn't, why hasn't it? If the athlete were to try the same intervention techniques again, what would have to change for the attempt to be successful? Can the athlete make the necessary changes? Can you convince him or her that it's worth a second try?

If the athlete is going to have faith in your recommendations, you will have to explain, in a very convincing way, why the outcome will be different this time. Do not make any recommendations until you know what the athlete has already tried.

8. Recommend specific steps that the athlete can be take to gain greater control over behavior.

One of the most difficult tasks for many service providers is to make realistic recommendations to their athletes. Your recommendations must fit the athlete's lifestyle, travel plans, and competition schedule. At professional and international levels, success is dictated by the bottom line. Here are some items to keep in mind, especially when working with elite-level athletes:

- Keep your recommendations focused on one issue or problem at a time.

- Keep the athlete's TAIS profile in mind as you make your recommendations. Based on TAIS scores, how much follow-through and personal responsibility can you expect the athlete to take? How easily will the athlete become overloaded and confused by your instructions?

- Make your recommendations as situation-specific as possible.

- Take advantage of any opportunity to involve others in the athlete's improvement plan. Use them to help provide support and to reinforce program keys. At the same time, be sensitive to any trust issues or concerns the athlete may have about providing information to others. You may inadvertently give someone else a competitive edge or cause a coach to lose confidence in the athlete.

- When possible, work with the coach and build any mental-skills training (e.g., concentration and arousal-control skills) into the athlete's practices.

- Time your interventions. Remember, any training that requires the athlete to consciously analyze and attend to new information during competition will disrupt performance for a while. Is the athlete's skill level and competition and practice schedule at a place where he or she can take that risk? Don't make changes just before a major competition.

- Once you have established a relationship with the athlete, take advantage of modern technology to stay in touch.

Numerous books offer information on mental-skills training techniques that you can use with athletes. Several of these are listed at the end of the chapter. Just remember to keep it simple; when it comes time to actually perform, most athletes need to stop thinking.

Using Role-Playing to Develop Your Skills

In our TAIS training and certification programs, the majority of the time is spent role-playing. We have found that this is the best way for people to quickly develop the skills they need to be comfortable and effective in feedback sessions.

Here's how we structure the role-playing situations: We divide the entire class into subgroups, with four people in each group. One member of each group plays the role of the athlete; another plays the role of the person providing feedback. The other two members are observer-coaches, one for the athlete and one for the person providing feedback. The roles change with each new case, so that everyone plays every role.

The profile of a case is projected onto a screen, and the entire group is given the same kind of information you were given about each of the cases in chapter 6. Group members are provided with a reason for testing and just enough information about the athlete to enable them to determine whether he or she has the technical skills required to perform. Next, each participant is asked to interpret the profile using the six-step process presented in chapter 6. Class members work alone and have from 15 to 20 minutes to complete this part of the assignment.

Once everyone has drawn his or her own conclusions based on the referral reasons and test information, the group breaks up into pairs. Each coach is paired with his or her respective partner. The athlete and the athlete coach work together to decide how to put on the profile and play the role during the feedback session. Their goal is to learn to translate test scores into actual interviewing behavior and to then act this out in the interview.

The individual providing feedback and the feedback coach also meet as a team, and their challenge is to anticipate how the athlete will behave during the interview and to answer the following questions:

- If the athlete behaves as the profile indicates, what can the person providing feedback expect to observe and encounter during the different stages of the feedback process?

- How should the interviewer behave during the interview, given the athlete's test profile? In other words, how can the interviewer use what he or she knows about the individual from the TAIS profile to increase the likelihood that he or she will be able to get relevant points across? Based on the person's profile, how controlling should the interviewer be, how much structure should the interviewer provide, how positive and supportive should the interviewer be, etc.?

The teams are given approximately 15 minutes to come up with their respective game plans, and then the interview begins. The interview lasts approximately 30 minutes. Given this limited time frame, we do not expect the interviewer to reach the recommendations stage.

During the interview, the coaches quietly observe the process. Each coach is allowed to call up to two time-outs during the role-playing. The time-outs should not last longer than 2 minutes. During the breaks, the coaches can comment on the process (e.g., how well the role-playing is going), provide support and encouragement (e.g., tell people what they are doing right), and offer one or two suggestions about techniques to try or other ways to behave.

An important point to keep in mind is that we don't script the role-play (other than to ask that the eight-step interview process be followed). In other words, we don't give the players a particular problem situation, nor do we tell them to cooperate, not to cooperate, etc. Instead, we are concerned with the process. Specifically, is the athlete able to understand and to get into the character as it is defined by the test scores? Is the interviewer able to anticipate the athlete's behavior? Does he or she follow the eight-step feedback process? We don't script, because real interviews aren't scripted. Comfort comes from knowing that you can reduce the unexpected in an interview by adequately anticipating and planning for some of the behaviors you will encounter. Comfort also comes from practicing and from having the opportunity to "go with the flow" in order to learn that adjustments can be made and that the unexpected can be dealt with effectively.

A good interview is like a good "at bat" in baseball. Even great hitters in baseball fail to get a hit 70% of the time (bat .300). Good hitting is not simply a matter of hits. Did the hitter swing at strikes and not swing at balls? Were the swings good ones? Did he or she make good contact with the ball? Judge the quality of the performance "at bat" and not just the outcome. Did the interviewer anticipate behavior? Were the responses appropriate? Were the right questions asked? When the process is good, the percentage of times the interviewer "hits" safely will increase, but he or she will never "bat a thousand."

Once the role-playing is finished, the whole class reassembles to discuss the process and to debrief. At this point, we talk about the specific recommendations we might make to help the athlete improve.

A Case Example

Let me use John, the sprinter, to illustrate the questions I formulated and the process I went through during our feedback session. I will also provide additional comments about the other eight cases presented in chapter 6.

Anticipating the Individual's Behavior Based on TAIS Scores

Although John was very willing to share his feelings of being overloaded (OIT), distracted (OET), depressed (DEP), and anxious (RED and OBS) on TAIS, I anticipated that it would be difficult to obtain information from him. His lack of confidence in his abilities to express himself (IEX) and to problem-solve (BIT) meant I would have to provide structure to get him to answer questions; that's what the test questions had done for him. I knew I would have to ask very specific questions to elicit the information from him. John would be confused by open-ended questions like "Tell me what you feel" or "Why do you think that's the case?" I had to stay away from "why" questions.

I also knew I would have to probe to make sure that any information John gave me was accurate and not just something he was saying to reduce the pressure he was feeling in the interview. I predicted that he might do this because on TAIS he indicated that he gets confused easily (OIT), is highly anxious (OBS), and doesn't like to argue (NAE and IEX). These qualities, combined with a tendency to withdraw (INT) and to agree with others to avoid conflict (PAE), suggested that John would be apt to agree with any interpretation I offered, just to get out of the room. My challenge was further complicated by the fact that I had been brought in by the coach.

In terms of the kind of performance errors John was likely to make, his relatively low level of self-confidence (SES), high level of introversion (INT), and tendency to ruminate and worry (OBS) suggested that he would frequently fail to react quickly enough. That he was also easily distracted (OET) and confused (OIT) and that he failed to make appropriate attentional shifts (RED) further complicated things. I hypothesized that growing pressure, from both internal and external sources, would inevitably force John to make decisions. When that happened, the decisions would not be well thought out and would seem impulsive to others; thus, John's pattern of error would be marked by inconsistency.

Establishing a Relationship

The hypothesis that John would not establish trust easily (INT, OBS) and the prediction that the harder I tried to establish a relationship, the more suspicion I would encounter, told me I should keep any introductions simple and to the point:

Hi, John. Thanks for responding to the inventory you were asked to fill out. I am going to provide you with some feedback based on your test scores, but before I do that I would like to tell you a little about myself and what the coach wants me to do. I would also like to find out from you how track is going and what it is that you're working on.

I work with professional and Olympic-level athletes in a number of different sports, helping them improve their ability to concentrate and helping them control the anxiety and frustration that sometimes get in the way of their ability to perform. Your coach has asked me to work with all of the sprinters who the United States believes have a chance at making the next Olympic team. The coach believes that what goes on in an athlete's head has a big impact on performance and he feels that I may be able to help each of you perform up to your full potential. That's a little bit about me. Do you have any questions?

Gathering Information About the Individual's Sport and Attitude Toward Testing

- *John, how long have you been running track?*

- *What's been the most difficult thing for you to learn?*

- *What do you enjoy most about running track?*

- *What are you trying to improve now?*

- *Are there any problems you are having that you think we should know about? For example, are you having any problems staying focused or concentrating?*

John's answers to these questions were predictably short and to the point. He had been running track for 10 years. The most difficult thing for him to learn was to stay down coming out of the blocks. What he enjoyed about running was the training and that he was good at it. Right now he was doing strength training, trying to get a little faster. He didn't have any problems that he thought I should know about.

To determine his attitude toward testing, or response set, I asked him, directly, how he was feeling when he responded to TAIS. Then, based on his responses, I offered an interpretation to see how he would react to it:

John, one of the things that is important when interpreting scores on the inventory you filled out is to find out about an athlete's attitude toward being asked to respond to the inventory. Do you remember what you were thinking or feeling as you answered the questions?

According to John, he was just trying to be honest and to do what was asked. He didn't know if it would help or not. I responded to that by saying,

I think you succeeded in being honest. In fact, you were much more honest than most athletes are when they answer the questions. Most athletes have a tendency to emphasize their strong points and minimize any weaknesses. You didn't do that. If anything, you may have been a little too hard on yourself, too critical. Do you think that's possible?

John's response was something like "I don't know. If you say so, I guess it could be."

At this point, I began to employ the eight steps for providing test feedback that are given in Table 6.

1. Describing

John, let me tell you what the inventory says about your concentration strengths and about how you get along with others. First, your scores agree with what the coach has told us about you. You've described yourself as extremely dedicated and hardworking, very focused on becoming better at your sport. That fits with what you told me you enjoy most about your sport—the training and the fact that you are good at it.

In addition, you've indicated that you are a good listener, more than willing to follow the advice that others give you. You are supportive of others and try to get along with everyone. Again, all of that fits with what your coach has told me about you, and it fits with the way you have interacted with me up to this point. Have I said anything that you would disagree with?

2. Educating

You know, in talking to your coach, I noticed that he couldn't think of anything about you that he would change. As far as he's concerned, you're the greatest. He really seems to love working with you. What's a little confusing to me is that your scores on TAIS suggest that you don't agree with the coach. You've indicated there are things that you would like to change. Can you tell me about those?

This question was too open-ended for John; he became visibly anxious and confused. He told me he didn't understand what I was asking. He didn't disagree with his coach, but he didn't disagree with me; he just didn't know. With that, he became silent.

John, your greatest strengths are your ability to focus your concentration, your willingness to work hard, to perfect the things you're good at. It's my experience that even for the greatest athletes in the world, their greatest strength, which—like yours—is their ability to focus concentration, can become their greatest weakness when they are under pressure.

You can become too focused and too dedicated. When that happens, you get too critical and demanding of yourself. You expect too much. That's what your scores on TAIS seem to indicate. If that's true, then when you get too critical, you stop focusing on the positive things—the things you can control—and start to focus on the negatives. You worry. You've described yourself as a quiet, agreeable guy, and you've indicated that you are very private and don't often share your feelings with others. As pressure increases, if you're like other world-class athletes with scores like yours, you'll become even quieter and share even less. If that's true, it's not surprising that your coach doesn't see you as having any problems or as being concerned about anything.

Your scores on the inventory tell me that you are being pretty hard on yourself, that you aren't feeling very happy about things. Are you willing to share some of your thoughts and feelings with me?

In response to this, John just said everything was fine with track and with the coach.

3. Empathizing

John, I believe you. I know that like you, the coach feels that everything is okay as far as he and track are concerned. But being both an athlete and a student can be pretty demanding, especially for someone who wants to do everything perfectly. Most of the athletes I know make their sport their priority, and schoolwork comes second. As long as they stay eligible, they don't worry about school. Your answers to the inventory indicate that you aren't comfortable with doing anything halfway. You worry about things. Are there things away from track and competition that are bothering you?

Like you, I'm a very private person. I don't find it easy to share my problems with others. Something inside me tells me that my problems are my responsibility, no one else can solve them for me. That inner voice makes it very hard to ask for help, because I am afraid others might think less of me if I do. I guess I've learned over the years that there are times when others can help. I believe this is one of them. I'd like to help, but I can't if you don't share the things that are bothering you.

4. Probing

This was enough to encourage John to begin talking about some of the pressure he was feeling. Throughout the process, however, I had to continue urging him to elaborate and to fill in details rather than to give vague, general answers.

5. Validating

John's behavior in the interview was consistent with his profile. The anxiety and confusion were there, as were the agreeableness and avoidance of confrontation. His introverted nature came through, as did his work ethic (in the content of what he said) and the high expectations he placed on himself. His interview behavior also validated his discomfort with abstract intellectual discussions and his lack of confidence in his ability to perform in an academic environment.

6. Assessing

The fact that John was honest on his test indicated he was trying to reach out for help. That I was able to get through to him enough to get him to talk about school and about home reinforced that prediction. Because the coach really cared about John, and because John was open to support and encouragement, there was hope.

7. Identifying

John had called his family and talked about leaving school and transferring to a college much closer to home. His mother didn't want him to do that. His education was important, and the academic and athletic programs of the school closer to home were not as strong. Other than that, John had not taken any steps to try to resolve his problems.

8. Recommending

My first step in this phase was to try to convince John to share his feelings with his coach. I was able to do that, but only by taking on much of the responsibility for talking to the coach. John wouldn't go on his own to talk with the coach, but he agreed to allow me to share with the coach some of the things that we had discussed.

I did some problem solving with the coach to determine the specific steps that could be taken to help John feel less isolated and more confident in school. The way to deal with John's avoidance of issues, and his ultimately impulsive decision making, was to help him to face them earlier while providing him with enough structure, direction, and support to enable him to control his anxiety.

Case 2—An Olympic Hopeful (Revisited)

Anticipating Pete's Behavior Based on TAIS Scores

Based on Pete's TAIS scores, I expected him to be very bright and very verbal (BIT, IEX). I also expected him to be extremely positive, competitive, and intellectually challenging (PAE, IEX). He would come to the interview well prepared and well organized (BIT, NAR), knowing what he wanted to say and knowing what he wanted from me. He would take control in the interview in a nice way, but take control nevertheless, directing the discussion where he felt it needed to go (CON, SES, and PAE). He would interrupt if things were moving too slowly or if he felt I needed help to keep up with his thinking. He would make up his mind very quickly as to whether or not he thought I could help.

Pete's scores on the TAIS scales measuring need for control (CON), self-confidence (SES), and physical competitiveness (P/O), along with his scores on intellectual expression (IEX), analytical thinking (IEX), and information processing (INFP), suggested that his most likely performance errors would result from overanalyzing. His scores also indicated that when he did overanalyze, he would become impatient (OBS) and frustrated with himself and his performance, although he would deny any real anger (NAE low).

Validating (Referral Question and TAIS Data)

Even before I interviewed Pete, many of his scores on TAIS appeared to be consensually validated by the information contained in the reason for referral. His analytical skills (BIT) and his ability to focus and discipline himself to organize and accomplish a goal (NAR) fit with his having built a company from the ground up (and having then quickly sold it for $30 million). This level of success appeared to justify his high level of self-confidence (SES), as well as his desire and willingness to take control (CON).

Case 3—Water Polo Madness (Revisited)

Anticipating Howard's Behavior Based on TAIS Scores

Based on Howard's TAIS scores, we expected him to scan his environment (BET) much of the time and to notice just about everything that went on during the interview, including any sounds from outside. He would react very quickly and confidently to questions (CON, SES). He would state exactly what was on his mind and have no problems sharing his feelings about others and about us (IEX, NAE, and PAE). Some of the positions he would take would not be well thought out (BCON, OBS, and low NAR). When challenged, he wouldn't back down; instead, he would continue to argue for his position, and his anger and frustration with us and with our questions would become obvious (BCON, NAE).

Howard's competitive mistakes would be a direct result of his loss of control over feelings of anger (BCON, NAE). Those feelings would be generated by a loss of control, by a failure on his part or on the part of the team to perform up to his expectations, or by confrontation and challenge from other players. Howard would react by becoming overly aggressive.

Validating (Referral Question and TAIS Data)

Information in the reason for referral provided consensual validation for many of Howard's TAIS scores. Certainly his scores on the behavior control scale (high BCON) and the negative affect expression scale (NAE) were consistent with the problems he was having; so, too, were his tendency to be more reactive than analytical (BET vs. BIT) and his speed when making decisions (low OBS).

Case 4—Gymnastics Superstar (Revisited)

Anticipating Ludmilla's Behavior Based on TAIS Scores

Ludmilla was an athlete who liked structure and was most comfortable when she could stay focused on one thing at a time (NAR, low INFP). She was a quiet individual with very little confidence in her analytical skills (IEX, BIT). Therefore, I would expect her to wait for me to take the lead in the interview. Her answers would be short and to the point, and I would have to ask many questions to get her to provide much detail, unless I focused on a single performance. If I asked her to describe her routine or her performance the last time she was on the uneven parallel bars, I anticipated that she would be capable of doing so with great attention to detail (NAR and OBS).

Ludmilla would avoid taking a firm position on anything she had even the smallest doubt about (OBS). When she would make a statement, I would expect her to qualify it (e.g., "Could be this, but . . . " or "Under these conditions I might . . . "). I thought she would become confused if I became too theoretical, but that she probably wouldn't tell me when that was happening (low IEX, NAE). The only way I'd be aware of her confusion would be by seeing a glazed or uncomfortable look in her eyes. I was probably going to have to ask her to repeat things or to paraphrase what I had said to make sure she had heard me accurately. I also knew that asking her to paraphrase things could generate considerable anxiety, especially if the point I had been trying to make was at all theoretical. I needed to watch for any anxiety that might develop when I pushed her to perform in an area where she lacked confidence.

From a performance perspective, Ludmilla's scores suggested she was a perfectionist, so I could expect her to be extremely hard on herself (NAR, RED, OBS, DEP). She would be prone to overtraining (NAR, RED, and OBS) and would have difficulty easing off just before a major competition. I might anticipate that Ludmilla would make very few errors, because she was a perfectionist competing in a sport that demands perfection. She would likely lack the ability to make adjustments quickly. Once she made a mistake during a routine, she would have a hard time forgetting about it and recovering (RED, OBS).

Validating (Referral Question and TAIS Data)

The information gained from the coach prior to testing appeared to validate many of Ludmilla's TAIS scores. Her focus, dedication, and attention to detail (NAR), as well as her concern about the avoidance of errors (high OBS), were certainly consistent with her level of performance and her sport. Her very low scores on the expressiveness scales—in particular, intellectual expression (IEX) and negative affect expression (NAE)—were also consistent with the coach's assertion that he still "didn't know her."

Case 5—Life on the Edge (Revisited)

Anticipating Heidi's Behavior Based on TAIS Scores (Include Type of Errors)

We predicted we would know that Heidi was arriving for her interview before we actually saw her. She would talk with others and impose herself on whatever was going on (EXT, BET, NAE, PAE, and low INT). As with Howard, we would expect Heidi to scan her environment almost constantly (BET). She would notice everything that went on during the interview, including any sounds from outside, and she would be reading us to see how we were responding to her. She would react very quickly and confidently to questions (CON, SES), stating exactly what was on her mind and easily sharing her feelings about others or about us (IEX, NAE, and PAE). When challenged, she would not back down; instead, she would continue to argue for her position, and her anger and frustration with us and with the questions would become obvious (BCON, NAE). If we pushed too hard, she would walk out of the interview.

We predicted that Heidi's competitive mistakes would result directly from a loss of control over her competitiveness (P/O) and from the anger that develops when she isn't winning and in control (CON, NAE, BCON). Interpersonally, Heidi would make the mistake of not listening to others (CON, SES) and of becoming so emotionally forceful in her presentations (NAE, PAE, BCON) that people would pay more attention to the emotional content of what she was communicating than to the intellectual content.

Validating (Referral Question and TAIS Data)

The coach's description of Heidi's behavior and his difficulty in working with her were consistent with her scores on the interpersonal side of the inventory

(CON, SES, NAE, and PAE). The hypothesis about the relationship between anger and Heidi's competitiveness and injury would have to be assessed in the interview. When questioning Heidi about that, we wanted to determine the extent to which her anger generated competitive intensity and the kind of focus that allowed her to ski fast without the excessive muscle tension that often develops when people try too hard. Heidi needed that focus, but it was also important that she keep her muscle tension from increasing too much. Her legs and hips had to be relaxed to take the bumps and to control her skis over the snow.

Case 6—The Moody Striker (Revisited)

Anticipating Sarah's Behavior Based on TAIS Scores

Sarah's behavior in the interview would likely depend on where she was in her menstrual cycle. Whether she was premenstrual or at midcycle, she would be interested in trying to learn more about herself (BIT, SES). If the appointment was just prior to the onset of menstruation, she would be more subdued, letting us do more of the talking and asking fewer questions (IEX, CON, P/O). She would also be less focused on what we were saying and more easily distracted by things going on around her (NAR, OET).

If we were interviewing Sarah midcycle, we would feel intellectually challenged, but not in a negative way, by someone who was extremely interested in everything we had to offer—someone who would challenge us to provide more information than we were prepared to give (BIT, NAR, INFP, IEX, SES, CON). We would probably find ourselves saying things like "I wish I could give you the answer to that" or "I'll have to try to find an answer to that for you."

Sarah's performance errors would also differ depending on where she was in her cycle. When she made a mistake midcycle, it would be because she was being too controlling, feeling too competitive, trying too hard, rushing, and getting frustrated (CON, SES, P/O, NAR). Just prior to menstruation, she would be more likely to become distracted both by things going on around her (OET) and by thoughts and feelings related to her perception of being out of control (CON, RED). She wouldn't have the same fire and energy for coping with distractions as she normally had (lower INFP, P/O, and CON). Thus, Sarah would shift from being too aggressive at times to not being aggressive enough.

Validating (Referral Question and TAIS Data)

Sarah's analytical skills (BIT), her desire to leave nothing to chance in preparation (NAR), her continual search for a competitive edge (P/O), her willingness to take the initiative (CON), and her self-confidence (SES) all appeared to be validated by both the reason for referral and the fact that Sarah had referred herself. Sarah was willing to confront any issue head-on and had obviously given some thought to what was happening.

Given Sarah's analytical skills and level of introspection, it was likely that in the interview she would consensually validate the differences between the two sets of TAIS scores. She knew herself and had described herself accurately (through her own eyes). Because we would see her under only one set of conditions, it would be difficult for us to ascertain whether the rather dramatic differences that existed on TAIS, and in Sarah's mind, were as obvious and dramatic to others. The only way to determine that would be to interview teammates, to observe Sarah over time, or to have someone who knew Sarah well respond to the inventory for her (using the same two response sets Sarah had used).

Suggested Readings

Dorfman, H. A., & Kuehl, K. (1989). *The mental game of baseball.* South Bend, IN: Diamond Communications.

Druckman, D., & Bjork, R. A. (Eds.). (1991). *In the mind's eye: Enhancing human performance.* Washington, DC: National Academy Press.

Fried, R. (1990). *The breath connection.* New York: Insight Books.

Jensen, P. (1992). *The inside edge.* Toronto: Macmillan.

Nideffer, R. M. (1992). *Psyched to win.* Champaign, IL: Leisure.

Nideffer, R. M. (1995). *Focus for success* (CD-ROM). San Diego, CA: Enhanced Performance Systems.

Reed, W. (1992). *A road that anyone can walk Ki.* Tokyo: Japan Publications.

Schmid, A., & Peper, E. (1998). Strategies for training concentration. In J. M. Williams (Ed.), *Applied sport psychology* (pp. 316–328). Mountain View, CA: Mayfield.

Selleck, G. A. (1995). *How to play the game of your life.* South Bend, IN: Diamond Communications.

Zinsser, N., Bunker, L., & Williams, J. M. (1998). Cognitive techniques for building confidence and enhancing performance. In J. M. Williams (Ed.), *Applied sport psychology* (pp. 270–295). Mountain View, CA: Mayfield.

Making Treatment Recommendations 8

There are many psychological intervention techniques that can be used to help athletes perform more effectively. Unfortunately, these techniques are often used inappropriately by coaches, athletes, and sport psychologists. Individuals become wedded to a particular technique and automatically apply it to every problem that is presented. They do this because they have a blind faith in the power of the technique. Hypnosis is frequently applied in this way. For many people, there remains something mystical, or magical, about hypnosis. They seem to believe that simple suggestions like "Perform better" or "Feel confident" will have the desired results merely because they are given while the subject is hypnotized. Other people misapply various psychological procedures because they have simplistic notions about the relationship between such features as an athlete's level of arousal and his or her performance. They also have simplistic notions about the ease with which training in the laboratory will generalize to an athlete's performance arena.

We know biofeedback clinicians who implicitly operate on the assumption that using biofeedback to learn to lower arousal will magically enable an athlete to perform better. For these individuals, low arousal is good and high arousal is bad. The same thing can be said about many other techniques often employed by sport psychologists. Progressive relaxation, autogenic training, cognitive techniques like mental rehearsal, visuo-motor behavior rehearsal, and rational emotive therapy often are applied in the same general way, to almost every situation, independent of the problem and sometimes independent of the athlete's basic concentration and interpersonal skills.

Before you automatically apply your technique of choice to the problem with which you are helping an athlete, ask yourself the following questions:

- Does the problem require major behavior change or simply fine-tuning?

- What specific kinds of behavior must be changed to improve performance?

- How will the technique(s) I intend to apply change those behaviors?

- How confident can I be that the learning that takes place will transfer to the actual performance situation?

- What will interfere with the athlete's adherence to the training program?

What is the difference between the athlete who uses anger to effectively motivate himself (and is seen as an intense competitor by others) and the athlete whose anger causes him to self-destruct (and is seen as a hothead or a loose cannon by others)? What is the difference between the athlete whose fear of making a mistake causes others to see her as highly focused and perfectionistic and the athlete whose fear of making a mistake causes others to see her as tentative and reluctant to take risks (someone who chokes under pressure)?

The difference lies in the frequency and intensity of the problems or mistakes that occur, rather than in the type of mistake. This is true for each kind of problem. Take anger, for example. If an athlete's anger is used effectively most of the time and helps him to perform, he will probably be labeled an intense competitor, and his occasional mistake will be tolerated. If, on the other hand, the anger frequently interferes with his performance, he will be labeled a hothead.

As a service provider in sport psychology, you will be asked to help individuals improve their performance. The frequency and intensity of the mistakes these individuals make will often result in their acquiring negative labels. If this has happened, the problem is likely to be severe enough that changes in the athlete's behavior will be necessary to correct it. At other times, however, you will be dealing with highly effective performers, individuals who are trying to fine-tune their performance and to reduce the frequency of their mistakes. For elite athletes, even one mistake at a crucial time is too many. Here you're talking not about behavior change, but about behavior management. Athletes from these two groups may make the same kind of mistakes, but you will treat them differently.

Consider two athletes, one who uses anger to perform more effectively and one who allows anger to interfere with effective performance. The level of motivation to change will differ dramatically for these two athletes. The athlete who is able to use anger effectively will be highly motivated to gain greater control but will resist making wholesale changes in behavior. Any intervention that fails to recognize the utility of this athlete's anger will be viewed with suspicion. Because fewer situations and stimuli will lead to the inappropriate expression of anger on the part of the "intense" athlete, interventions should be much more situation-specific than they would be for the "hotheaded" athlete. The less control the athlete has over his or her expression of anger, the more likely it is that weaknesses in several areas (building blocks) are contributing to the problem and that you will have to involve others (e.g., coaches and teammates) in the helping process.

What Are the Specific Behaviors That Have to Change to Improve Performance?

In chapter 6, we talked about how to use results from TAIS to (a) predict the types of problems an athlete is liable to have and (b) identify the specific concentration, intrapersonal, and interpersonal skills that would have to change for improved performance. In the next few paragraphs, we will use the data from Case 3 in chapter 6 to talk about the changes that Howard, our water polo player, must make to gain control over his anger. While reviewing Howard's profile, we'll also point out some of the differences between his scores and those of other individuals who have anger issues.

Howard's profile typifies the profile of an athlete who has problems controlling anger. From a concentration standpoint, his highest score is on the scale measuring environmental awareness and the ability to react quickly and instinctively to the environment (BET). This particular focus is much more likely to contribute to an outward expression of anger than is either an analytical focus (BIT) or a narrow focus (NAR) of concentration. A broad-external focus of concentration contributes to a loss of control in two ways. First, heavy reliance on this ability prevents some of the early analysis that might help an athlete like Howard recognize a buildup in emotional arousal. As arousal increases, loss of control becomes more likely. Second, this broad focus of concentration increases the athlete's awareness of behavior that is irritating. When concentration narrows and zooms in on the source of the irritation, control is lost.

On the interpersonal side, an individual who desires to be in control (CON), who is competitive (P/O) and self-confident (SES), and who makes quick decisions (low OBS) is likely to make the kind of mistakes associated with being overly assertive and overly competitive. The higher such an athlete scores on the behavior control scale (high BCON means less impulse control) and on negative affect expression (NAE), the more frequent and intense the emotional expressions of anger are likely to be.

As you can see, almost everything in Howard's profile seems to contribute in one way or another to his loss of control over anger. So what do you change to help him gain greater control over his behavior?

- Would Howard's problem be so pervasive and intense if he scored higher on the analytical scale (BIT)?

- Would it be as pervasive and intense if he scored higher on the scale measuring a narrow focus (NAR)?

- Would Howard's anger be as likely to be externally directed if he scored lower on the self-esteem scale (SES) or lower on the negative affect expression scale (NAE)?

- Would Howard's loss of control be as pervasive and intense if his speed of decision making (OBS) were slower or if he had a lower score on the behavior control scale (BCON)?

- Would Howard's loss of control over anger be as frequent if his scores on the control scale (CON) and the competitiveness scale (P/O) were lower?

The answer to all of these questions is no. Changes in any of those variables would help Howard to better control his anger. The question is, do you want to make changes in some of these variables? You don't want to stop him from being competitive or from wanting to take control of situations. If you made changes in those characteristics, the cure might be worse than the problem.

To control his anger more effectively, Howard must retain control over his ability to shift his focus of concentration so he can anticipate the consequences of his actions. This will enable him to see the whole pool. Additionally, he must prevent his muscle tension from increasing to a point where it interferes with his performance. What techniques would you use to help Howard, and how would these affect his ability to shift concentration and to maintain control over muscle tension? What other characteristics would be affected by the intervention, and what impact would that have on Howard's performance?

How Will the Techniques We Apply Change Relevant Behavior?

Almost any relaxation technique might bring about a positive change in Howard's behavior. Increased relaxation would broaden his attention and reduce in his level of muscle tension. Because Howard has the technical and tactical skills required to perform effectively (when he controls his focus of concentration and his level of muscle tension), anything that reduces his emotional arousal should help.

During competition, Howard does not have much time to relax; yet from a performance standpoint, this is when he needs relaxation the most. What relaxation techniques can you teach Howard to use in the performance setting? Perhaps more important, how can you help Howard to recognize when relaxation is necessary? When the importance of the competition is building, and the play grows rougher, will Howard remember to calm down? Not if his past behavior is any indication. How can you adapt techniques like mental rehearsal, visual-motor behavior rehearsal, or attention-control training to help Howard remember to relax early enough in the competition to make a difference? How do you get the techniques that Howard practices away from the pool, outside of the actual competition, to apply to the performance situation?

We would bring Howard into the office, explain to him why he's losing control, and point out how learning to relax just a little can help him maintain his ability to see everything that is happening in the pool. We would promise to help him maintain control over his anger to focus it, so that he can be more effective as a competitor. We would explain the link between experiencing excessive anger and trying too hard, pointing out how muscle tension increases and how that can affect his passes and his swimming skills.

We would teach Howard how to use autogenic training procedures to quickly develop feelings of relaxation, or we might teach him to use brief relaxation techniques, such as centering or alert hypnosis, to quickly relax. We would use a relaxation technique like progressive relaxation biofeedback or hypnosis to help Howard relax in the office, so that he can take full advantage of mental-rehearsal procedures and suggestions we might make. With Howard relaxed, we would have him mentally rehearse competitions. We would focus on increasing his self-awareness in order to make him more sensitive to increased emotional arousal, and we would build in a rehearsal of the relaxation techniques Howard would use in the actual situation.

Would all of this work? Would this be the best way to work with Howard? Would it be cost-effective? How long would you have to work with Howard to have a positive effect? How much time do you have? Would you need to do all of those things? Would you need to do more?

Let's look at some of the very practical problems associated with the treatment program we just outlined. First, it will require many sessions to be effective. It can take 6 months of daily practice for a person to learn to use autogenic training effectively. Do you have the luxury of seeing Howard every day? If you see him only once or twice a week, it is not likely that you will bring about the changes the coach wants to see (by the next competition).

Athletes have to overlearn physical skills to be able to execute them under pressure. Students have to overlearn problem-solving skills to be able to execute them under pressure. Howard is no different. He will have to overlearn any rehearsal and relaxation technique you teach him if he expects to remember to use it effectively. This will take self-discipline and time.

Look at Howard's TAIS profile. Does he have the self-discipline necessary to accept responsibility for himself, to practice the required procedures as often and as intensely as he will need to? Probably not. He is naturally gifted but is not particularly disciplined (NAR is low; BCON is high), and he has an inflated opinion of himself and his abilities (SES). Even if he is momentarily convinced that he has a problem, it won't be long before he will think he has the problem beaten and will stop practicing.

How long would it take you to teach Howard to behave with more self-discipline? If our longitudinal studies are any indication, even after a year of training designed to help him become more focused (higher NAR), you would be unlikely to see more than a 2% to 5% change in Howard's score (Nideffer, Sagal, Lowry, & Bond, 2000). If you did see dramatic changes, wouldn't that diminish something else? Wouldn't Howard become less capable of reacting instinctively?

We have no doubt that if you could get Howard to spend a couple of hours each day mentally rehearsing competitive situations in great detail, he would gain greater control and become a better player. Unfortunately, Howard is not the kind of athlete who will devote this kind of time to the development of his skills. He's too extroverted, too reactive to the environment (BET), and too impulsive (BCON). He also lacks the necessary focus and follow-through (NAR).

What can you do, given the constraints placed on you by the competitive environment, by the coach, and by Howard's attentional and interpersonal characteristics? Here is what we would suggest:

- Educate Howard about the effects that increasing emotional arousal has on his focus of concentration and on his muscle tension. Show how his strengths—his sensitivity to the environment and his competitiveness—turn into weaknesses at critical times.

- Teach Howard a brief relaxation technique such as centering or deep breathing—something he can use in a competitive situation. Have him identify appropriate times during competition when he can use the technique (e.g., when it won't interfere with the flow of the competition).

- Enlist the support of the coach and of Howard's teammates. Build your simulation training into team practice. Assign someone the responsibility of trying to cause Howard to lose control. Assign someone else the responsibility of signaling Howard and reminding him to use the relaxation procedure to broaden his focus. For example, the goalie or the athlete who is about to pass the ball to Howard may use a signal or a word to remind him to take a deep breath. Get the coach and teammates to serve as positive reinforcers for Howard when he does use the procedure.

Under the above conditions, you won't make any changes in Howard's basic personality or in the way he processes information. Howard will not gain much control over his behavior, but he may learn to recognize and to admit his weaknesses. He may also realize that he can use others to help him control and compensate for weaknesses. Without this environmental engineering, he will continue to make the same mistakes. If you were to move him to another team, or into another competitive arena, the same problems would occur.

It is conceivable that the success Howard may experience with the help of his teammates would ultimately lead to his willingness to make some personal sacrifices in order to gain greater self-control. His success, and the success of the team, might be reinforcement enough to motivate him to devote time to developing greater self-discipline and self-control. If this happens, other aspects of his behavior might change. He might become less extroverted and more introverted (something that frequently happens as athletes become more skilled and older). He might also begin to take more time to make decisions (OBS). He might even become more focused, more analytical, and a little less reactive.

Suggested Readings

Nideffer, R. M., Sagal, M. S., Lowry, M., & Bond, J. (in press). Identifying and developing world class performers. In G. Tennenbaum (Ed.), *The practice of sport and exercise psychology: International perspective.* Morgantown, WV: Fitness Information Technology, Inc.

Suinn, R. (1993). Imagery. In R. N. Singer, M. Murphey, & L. K. Tennant (Eds.), *Handbook of research on sport psychology* (pp. 492–510). New York: Macmillan.

Williams, J. M. (1998). *Applied sport psychology.* Mountain View, CA: Mayfield.

Writing Reports to Other Professionals

9

There are times when we are asked to provide others with our professional opinion about an athlete or a coach. Such a request typically comes from an individual who is responsible either for making an important decision about the athlete (e.g., whether to draft the athlete or not) or for overseeing the athlete's development and performance. Before we can agree to provide that kind of report, we must assure ourselves that

- the athlete has been informed about how test results will be used and is willing to have us provide a report,

- the information contained in the report will not violate any privilege of confidentiality we have with the athlete, and

- the individual to whom we are providing the report will use the information in a responsible and ethical manner.

Ensuring that the individual to whom we provide a report will use it ethically and responsibly is the biggest challenge. Frequently, we give reports to coaches or managers who have little formal training in psychology and, as a result, have extremely limited knowledge about issues relating to validity and reliability. For that reason, we use care in presenting our findings and opinions. In this chapter, we will cover some of the do's and don'ts of report writing. We have two goals we hope to accomplish with this chapter:

1. We want to sensitize you to key issues as you write your report.

2. We want to provide you with a general structure that you can use as a guide when writing reports that will be given to a third party.

Issues to Keep in Mind When Writing a Report

The last thing you need to worry about when you write a report is that it will not be taken seriously; instead, you should be concerned that it might be taken too seriously. The individual who takes your report too seriously will fail to ask questions, will suspend his or her own judgment, and will take what you say on blind faith. Do your best to ensure this does not happen. Your report will be based on very little information. The people who read it need to make sure that the statements you make and the conclusions you draw are accurate; write your report in a way that encourages them to do so.

Here are some general rules we believe increase the likelihood that others will use what you write in responsible and ethical ways:

- Don't use psychological jargon. If you can't say something that anyone with an eighth-grade education could understand, don't say it.

- Don't include raw test information or any kind of information (e.g., a test profile) when you have doubts about the individual's ability to understand it. Do, however, let the individual know the different types of information you evaluated and describe how they relate behaviorally to any conclusions you've drawn.

- Don't overgeneralize. Keep your report focused on a particular issue (e.g., the reason for referral) or performance situation. Do describe the conditions under which the data were collected and make a statement about your belief in the accuracy of the data. Make it clear that your interpretations are focused on, and limited to, the specific referral issue.

- Don't apply labels to behaviors (e.g., choking), but do describe what is going on, using actual behaviors that have been, or can be, observed. Also, describe the specific conditions most likely to lead to success for the individual, as well as those most likely to cause problems.

- Don't make decisions for others. Instead, articulate the different options and identify the issues and risks that must be considered with each option.

Don't Use Psychological Jargon.

The more highly trained you are, the harder it will be for you to follow this suggestion. To the highly trained professional, psychological jargon becomes a useful shorthand for communicating fairly complicated information. Professionals in sport psychology become so accustomed to terms like *normative data, consensual validation, mean,* and *standard deviation* that using them becomes second nature. If you are fortunate enough to have a secretary or someone else who types your reports, you can ask that person to help alert you to any technical terms or jargon that might make its way into your report. If you do your own typing, try to read the report from the perspective of someone who lacks any in-depth psychological knowledge.

Don't Include Raw Test Information.

Unless an individual has read and understands the test manuals that describe the validity and reliability of the inventory, he or she will not be able to responsibly use raw test data (e.g., the answers the subject gives to individual test items) or the summary information contained in most test profiles.

Don't Overgeneralize.

One of the biggest concerns we have when we provide feedback to third parties is that they will take out of context what we say about the individual who has been tested and that they will then overgeneralize. For example, we may indicate in a report that X is more of a team leader than a team player. We don't want the person reading the report to jump to the general conclusion that the individual tested is "not a team player."

Our interpretation is actually based on several factors. It is based on (a) the scores of the subject on test scales measuring characteristics such as the need to be in control or to be in a leadership position, (b) our understanding of the individual's level of motivation to succeed within a particular performance environment, (c) what we know about the people with whom the individual will be interacting (e.g., coaches, teammates), and (d) our understanding of the demands of a particular performance setting or situation. We must communicate to the person who reads our report that all of these factors play a role in the conclusions we are drawing. The best way to make that clear is to describe the specific conditions under which we believe the individual will feel a strong need to be a leader, as opposed to being a follower.

Don't Apply Labels; Avoid Using Terms That Are Emotionally Charged.

As a professional, you may have a very clear behavioral definition for a term like *choking*. To you, choking is an athlete's response to a specific set of performance conditions. When choking occurs, the athlete's focus of concentration narrows and centers on internal thoughts and feelings. This kind of focus makes it difficult, if not impossible, to perform. It leads to mistakes that act to increase anxiety and arousal, which, in turn, increase the number of mistakes the athlete makes. Performance goes from bad to worse. As a professional, you recognize that according to the above definition, under the right set of circumstances even the best performers in the world can choke.

Because you have a very clear, behaviorally objective definition of the term, you can use it effectively; you are not likely to overgeneralize or to label the athlete in a negative or unfair way. When you see the term being used, it signals you to identify the specific conditions that contribute to the downward performance spiral.

Unfortunately, choking is a term that most people use as a more general label to describe an individual who is unable to perform in any pressure situation. To them, a choker is a "head case," someone with a serious problem. These people overgeneralize when they hear the word "choke." They draw unfair and inaccurate inferences about the individual and his or her ability to perform. That is why it is important to take the time to describe the behavior within a situational context. For instance:

> "John's desire to perform well, combined with worry about letting the team down, caused his muscles to tighten up and prevented him from picking up the ball as quickly as he needed to. As a result, he didn't get around on the pitch and didn't perform as well as he would have liked. His failure in that at bat was still bothering him the next time he went to the plate, and as a result, he performed poorly again."

Putting John's behavior into a situational context makes it understandable and gives him hope. We can do something about the problem if we can reduce John's worry and control his tension. Saying that John choked doesn't provide him with any hope or direction.

Don't Make Decisions; Describe Conditions for Success and Failure.

As a sport psychologist, you are regarded as an expert within a particular area. Your job is to provide information from your area of expertise. The data you provide should never be the sole criteria for making a critical decision about someone. Coaches and managers, like all people, become emotionally involved with the people they work with. It isn't easy for them to say no to someone they like. It isn't easy for them to fire someone who they know is working just as hard as he or she can, someone who really cares, someone who is loyal to them and to the organization.

The pressure that decision makers are under often causes them to seek an escape hatch, a way out. You will undoubtedly find yourself in positions in which decision makers are asking you to do their job for them. Although it may be appropriate for you to empathize with their difficulty, it is not appropriate for you to assume their role. Consider the following:

You have been asked to assess an individual to provide information that will be used to make a decision about whether or not he should be drafted. The referral question may have been something like "We want to know if this individual has the psychological characteristics required for success."

Upon testing the athlete, you feel that he does not have the psychological characteristics required for success, and you are tempted to say just that: "Don't draft him. He lacks self-discipline and won't fit in." What is wrong with this statement?

Your statement is based on some very specific data and upon assumptions that you are making about the organization and its resources (e.g., coaches, etc.). Your assumptions may or may not be correct. Unless you make those assumptions explicit, the person who is responsible for making the decision can neither consensually validate nor invalidate them.

To illustrate the point, an individual who lacks self-discipline can be successful in a highly controlling organization, provided he or she is willing to submit to those organizational controls. In this case, the organization provides the discipline. In the example provided above, an assumption was made that the organization could not, or would not, provide that kind of control. Unfortunately, that assumption was not made explicit. It would have been much better to define the requirements of success, then to allow the decision maker to determine whether or not the organization could meet those requirements.

Sample Report

The following report is fairly typical of the reports we write and submit to third parties. In this particular case, the report was being sent to the head of player development for a professional franchise. This was an individual we had worked with before, someone who we knew had the interests of the athlete at heart. The purpose of the report was to define the conditions that would maximize the likelihood that this athlete would fulfill his potential.

To help you understand our conclusions, we have included a copy of the athlete's TAIS profile. Specific scale references were omitted in the report that went to the head of player development.

Psychological Report

Name: J   Date: October 1998

Job: Professional Athlete   Organization: ----------

Source and Reason for Referral

J was referred for an evaluation by the head of player development for the Illinois Rockets, John Smith. Mr. Smith described J as an extremely talented 20-year-old athlete who has not developed as the organization had hoped. From Mr. Smith's perspective, J would become easily frustrated when he wasn't performing up to his own expectations. When that would happen, J's performance would begin a downward slide and usually end up with J exploding. Recently, J's progress had been slowed down even more by a very serious injury that was the direct result of his driving recklessly while under the influence of alcohol.

While speeding to get away from a group of individuals who were chasing him, J ran into the back of a truck that had pieces of lumber sticking out. One of the two-by-fours went through the front window and struck J just above his right eye. He was hospitalized for an extended period of time and underwent both plastic surgery to reconstruct his face and surgery on his eye to correct damage done by the impact. J's recovery from surgery was just about complete, and his doctors had given him permission to "slowly" begin actual training for his sport.

At the time of testing and our interview with him, J was involved in a court-mandated alcohol rehabilitation program. Mr. Smith and the team had a great deal invested in J and were interested in gaining any information that J could use, or the team could use, to help J reach his full potential as an athlete.

Behavioral Observations

Because he had his driver's license taken away as a result of his accident, J's mother brought him to the interview. J came across as a very outgoing, cooperative, and highly motivated individual. He indicated that he realized he had made a serious mistake and said that it wouldn't happen again: "I owe too much to my dad." J's father had passed away the previous year and had devoted his life to helping his son develop as an athlete. J felt that he had let his father down.

The idea of testing was introduced to J as a means of identifying his performance strengths and weaknesses. He knew both testing and the interviews we would be conducting would provide him and the head of player development with information we believed would help him live up to his potential as an athlete.

Test Administered and Results

The Attentional and Interpersonal Style (TAIS) Inventory

TAIS is a 144-item paper-and-pencil inventory that examines an athlete's concentration and communication skills, as well as his or her level of motivation and self-discipline. On TAIS, J described himself as an extremely competitive (P/O) and confident individual (SES) who likes the challenges associated with taking control and assuming responsibility (CON). He indicated that he is very sensitive to his environment and to the moods and feelings of others (BET). He described himself as a person who likes being with others (EXT), and as someone who is very positive and supportive (PAE). J also indicated that he has a tremendous amount of energy and becomes easily bored (INFP, OBS). J does not find it easy to do the same things over and over again. He's not an athlete who enjoys paying attention to details (NAR).

Based on our knowledge of J's failure to live up to his potential to this point and based on the problems his drinking has caused, his test scores appear to be much higher and more positive than we would expect. This suggests that J was somewhat naive and insensitive to his weaknesses and limitations. This interpretation appears consistent with our discussions with J about his accident.

When we confronted J about his mistakes, he readily admitted them. When we asked how he would prevent similar mistakes from occurring in the future, however, he seemed genuinely puzzled. His response was, "I've seen what can happen, and I won't do it again." Try as we might, we couldn't seem to get him to recognize that he might not be able to rely on willpower alone to keep him from getting into trouble. In his mind, that was all it would take: "I want to be successful, and I don't want to let my father down."

In our discussions with J, he indicated that he was a real extrovert and loved to "go out dancing and hang out with friends." When we suggested that those activities might get in the way of training and practice or lead to problems with alcohol, he denied it. "No, my friends want me to be successful. They'll keep me out of trouble."

Summary and Recommendations

J is a highly talented athlete who has failed to develop as quickly as everyone had hoped. Although highly energetic, positive, and enthusiastic, J appears to lack some of the self-discipline (NAR, OBS, moderate EXT) that most elite athletes have.

It may be that J's tremendous physical assets have compensated for a relative lack of self-discipline. It may also be that J's father provided the structure and direction his son needed in the past, and now that is gone. This particular interpretation would be at least partially supported by the fact that J emphasized numerous times that he was the man of the house now, and he had to take care of his mother and sister.

J's pattern of scores and his unrealistic perception of his own abilities are consistent with the tendency to become frustrated when things aren't going as planned. For a long time, he was so physically gifted relative to the competition that he had no concept of failure. Now, with a leveling in the playing field, he is experiencing much more pressure, and he doesn't have many coping skills. Thus far, J appears to be reacting to failure and frustration by telling himself that he is better than the results indicate; that he has talent; and that if he wants to succeed badly enough, he'll be successful. To J, however, wanting it badly enough means believing in himself and his potential; it doesn't mean working hard and making personal sacrifices.

It does not appear to us, at least at this time, as though J has the self-discipline necessary to take independent responsibility for his development. For J to achieve his potential, he will need considerable support and direction from management.

J's need for and enjoyment of social involvement, combined with the fact that he is easily bored, mean that he can be relatively easily distracted. When that happens, he "gets into the moment" and loses some of his ability to monitor his own behavior and prevent himself from getting into trouble. Who J rooms with and associates with when he is with the team will be very important. He needs good role models, individuals with self-discipline, individuals who can own both their strengths and their weaknesses, individuals who can accept direction and support from others when it is needed. J still needs others to provide some of the structure and direction his father provided for him before his father's death. Because he is highly motivated and because he wants to please his family, J is highly likely to accept any structure and support that are offered. Just make sure that this structure and support will lead in the direction of actualizing his potential.

With respect to the pressure that he puts on himself and the associated

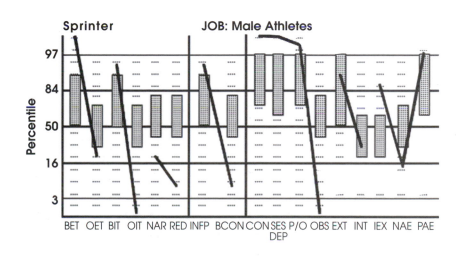

TAIS PERCENTILE SCORES

Name: J   **Norms/Rating: Male Athletes**

Attentional Characteristics	You	Norms	Interpersonal Style	You	Norms
External Awareness	99	70	Extroverted/Outgoing	88	75
External Distractibility	25	50	Introverted/Private	30	45
Analytical/Conceptual Skill	93	68	Intellectually Competitive	83	45
Internal Distractibility	2	50	Confrontive/Express Anger	17	50
			Supportive/Encouraging	95	80
Ability to Narrow Focus	25	60	Self-Critical	1	35
Breakdown in Shifting Focus	7	55			

Behavior Control	You	Norms
Energy Need for Diversity	93	70
Impulsive/Nonconforming	7	60

Interpersonal Style	You	Norms
Need for Control/Leadership	99	88
Self-Esteem/Confidence	99	83
Physically Competitive	98	90
Speed of Decisions/Worry	2	60

loss of control over his feelings of frustration and anger, J could benefit from some psychological skill building. This would involve working with the coaching staff as well as working with J. Consultation with the coaching staff would be necessary to identify the specific situations that cause problems for J, to target the intervention, and to help J establish realistic goals. Once a program to help J control his emotions has been designed and is in place, it will require the support and reinforcement of the coaching staff to ensure that J follows through.

Summary and Conclusions

In this chapter, we identified some of the ethical and practical issues to bear in mind when writing assessment reports for someone other than the person tested. You must maintain confidentiality, and the individual tested has a right to know what you will be saying in your report. It is our practice to go over the main areas of the report with the individual before it is sent out. This provides an opportunity for us to ensure that we do have the person's cooperation, and it provides a final opportunity to consensually validate our findings and conclusions.

There should be little disagreement around issues of confidentiality and the withholding of information that might be used inappropriately (e.g., raw test data or test profiles that require special knowledge to interpret). There may, however, be other areas in which you question our actions or conclusions. Perhaps we can point out a couple that you might want to think about and discuss with others:

- It became obvious in our discussions with J that his father had played a major role in his life and that the death of his father was something he was still dealing with. In spite of this fact, we chose not to become involved in counseling or therapy with J at the time. It is conceivable that the death of his father was playing a role in J's problems and would ultimately have an impact on his future development. Would you have handled this differently? If so, why? If not, why not?

- In our recommendations, we indicated that J could benefit from psychological-skill building to gain greater control over his anger and frustration. We provided some information about the type of involvement we would need from the organization, but we didn't go into great detail. Our strategy was to generate interest that would lead to more in-depth discussion. Would you have handled this differently?

Evaluating Psychological Tests

10

Establishing the validity and reliability of the inventories you employ is an important responsibility. This requires a basic understanding of *correlational statistics*, because they are used extensively in the research literature. As this book deals with assessment rather than with statistics, our goal here is to provide enough understanding about correlational data for you to become competent at evaluating research on psychological tests.

What Is a Correlation Coefficient?

Correlational statistics, whether the result of simple correlation coefficients or more complex calculations like regression equations, factor analysis, and multidiscriminate function analysis, provides the foundation for establishing the validity and the reliability of psychological tests. On the basis of studies employing these statistical techniques, conclusions are drawn about the utility, validity, and reliability of psychological tests. A *correlation coefficient* is simply a number between −1.0 and +1.0 that indicates the strength of the relationship between two sets of numbers. While this is a relatively simple and straightforward description, there is more to correlational statistics than correlation coefficients.

Amount of Variance Accounted For

If you want to find out if body weight has a tendency to increase along with height (weight and height are two different variables represented by numbers), the correlation coefficient, a simple statistic, will allow you to see if the two are related. You can also find out whether a group of students' scores on a midterm exam are related to their scores on the final. The correlation coefficient will tell you if those students who had the highest scores on the midterm also had them on the final.

The Venn diagrams shown in Figure 10 can help you see how the size of the correlation coefficient provides an indication of the strength of the relationship between two variables. The stronger the relationship, the more effectively you can use one set of scores to predict the other.

As we have said, correlation coefficients range in value from −1.0 to 1.0. The nature of the relationship between the two sets of scores is determined by the sign of the correlation coefficient. If the score is negative, then a high

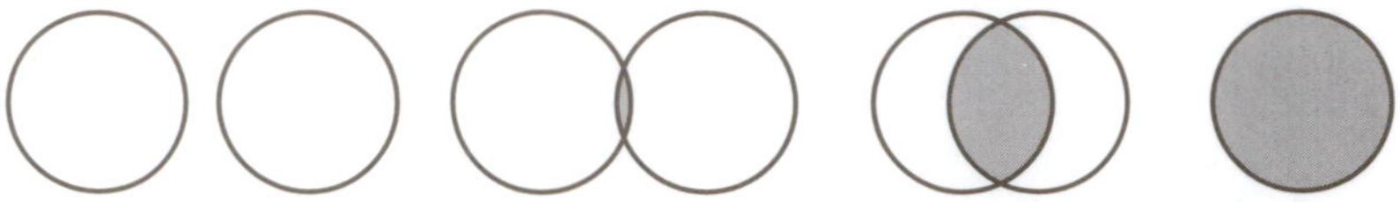

$r_{xy} = 0.0$ $r_{xy} = 0.3$ $r_{xy} = 0.7$ $r_{xy} = 1.0$

Figure 10. Amount of variance accounted for.

score on one set of numbers is associated with a low score on the other. If the score is positive, then a person who scores high on one set of numbers will also score high on the second set. To calculate the degree of predictability or overlap between two events, you simply square the correlation coefficient. Statisticians refer to the square of a correlation as *the amount of variance accounted for.*

Think about a correlation between a group of student scores on a midterm and corresponding student scores on the final. If the correlation were 0.0, there would be no overlap at all and, thus, no predictable relationship. Knowing a student's score on the midterm would not tell you anything about how he or she scored on the final. Some of the students who had low scores on the midterm would have high scores on the final; some who had high scores on the midterm would have low scores on the final; some would stay the same. If the correlation were .71, the square of the correlation would be .50, and you would have a 50% overlap between the two sets of scores. If the .71 correlation were positive, then most of the students who had a high score on the midterm would have a high score on the final. If the correlation were negative, then most of the students scoring high on the midterm would have scored low on the final. Finally, if the correlation were a plus or minus 1.0, the two distributions of scores would overlap completely. If you knew a student's score on the midterm, you could predict his or her score on the final, and vice versa. The correlation coefficient in this case accounts for, or explains, all of the variability (variance) in the scores.

Statistical Significance

To protect researchers from concluding that the correlational relationships found are reliable and are not simply due to chance, special statistical tables have been constructed. These tables are based on the number of subjects included in the study and have a dramatic effect on the size of the correlation required before it is considered *statistically significant.* For example, if you had collected data on a total of 8 subjects, you would need to obtain a correlation of .71 before you could conclude that your results were not due to chance. Remember this: A correlation of .71 would account for 50% of the variance. If you had collected data on a total of 100 subjects, you would only have to obtain a correlation of .20 before you could conclude that your results were not due to chance. A correlation of .2, when squared, accounts for only 4% of the variance. With 100 subjects, you would have a statistically significant finding, but knowing how a subject scored on one variable would not really allow you to predict his or her score on the second with much accuracy (less than 4%).

How Correlations Are Used

A correlation tells you how strongly two sets of numbers are related to one another. If the two sets of numbers are related in a statistically significant way, and if they account for a large amount of variance, then knowing how an individual scored on one measure will enable you to predict how he or she scored on the second.

One of the goals in sport psychology is to be able to predict the performance of athletes. You want to acquire this skill for two reasons: (a) to identify the athletes who are most likely to be successful and (b) to provide additional training to those who are less likely to be successful.

As a practitioner, you have probably noticed that the athletes who seem most successful to you are the hardest workers, the ones who are willing to sacrifice the most, the ones who take the time to perfect their skills, and the ones who rehearse their performance.

Let's say that you decide to develop a questionnaire to measure an athlete's ability to stay focused. You create a 10-item questionnaire with items like "I spend more time thinking about my sport and mentally rehearsing my performance than do most of the athletes I know." The subject responds to each of the items on the questionnaire by selecting one of the following options: "never," "rarely," "sometimes," "frequently," and "always." You assign numbers to the subjects' responses: "never" = 1; "rarely" = 2, "sometimes" = 3; "frequently" = 4; and "always" = 5. The scores subjects can obtain by responding to your 10-item questionnaire will range from 10 (for all "never" responses) to 50 (for all "always" responses).

Internal Consistency

You certainly want to demonstrate that each of the items in your questionnaire measures the same construct (i.e., commitment and focus). One way of establishing the internal consistency of your measure is to correlate each of the items contained in the inventory with the subject's total score on the inventory or scale. This is important because each of the items you have developed is assumed to measure the same construct, but from a slightly different angle. If the items are measuring the same construct and are contributing in a reliable way to the total score, they should be correlated with that score.

You administer the inventory to 100 subjects and then compute correlation coefficients that compare each of the items to the total score. With 100 subjects, a table of correlation coefficients indicates that your correlation must be .20 or higher to be statistically significant. Your analysis reveals that all of your correlations are significant and that they range from .35 to .80.

Test-Retest Reliability

Next, you must determine the test-retest reliability of your inventory. If you administer the test to the same 100 subjects after 2 weeks, will they score the same? How stable do you expect the construct of focus to be over time? If you anticipate that the characteristic is very stable and traitlike, you would expect a very high correlation between subject scores on the first test and scores on the second test. On the other hand, the more you think that learning and various situational factors can influence the construct, the lower the correlation you would expect.

You administer the test a second time, a year later. The correlation you get between subject scores on the first test and scores on the second is .81. A correlation of .81 accounts for about 65% of the variance. You conclude that the construct of focus is traitlike, stable over time and across situations.

Validity

You have an internally consistent and reliable measure, but does it really measure what you have designed it to measure? Do you have a valid instrument? One of the ways to check is to look at the items and see if they appear to be logically related to the construct you are measuring. If they do, then you have a *face-valid* measure. This is one important type of validity. There are other types that are at least as important—*construct validity* and *predictive validity*. One way to establish construct validity is to show that the scores on your inventory are correlated with other measures of the same construct (assuming that some exist). Therefore, you go to the testing literature and search for other inventories that might measure your construct, the ability to focus. You come across the digit-span subtest on the Wechsler Adult Intelligence Scale. The test measures how many numbers an individual can remember. One of the attributes the digit-span subtest is presumed to measure is an individual's ability to sustain attention and focus.

You get a group of 30 college students and administer both your test and the digit-span test to them. You then compute a correlation between subject scores on both tests. The correlation you obtain is .31. You check the statistical tables and find that you need a correlation of .35 to be sure that the relationship between the two tests is statistically significant.

You are about to conclude that the two instruments may not be measuring anything in common and are not predictably related, when someone points out that the digit-span subtest was validated on the general population, not on a college population. This individual tells you that college students tend to be more focused than noncollege students and, as a result, score much higher than does the average person in the population on the digit-span test. You look at the scores for your subjects and find that indeed, they are all fairly high. The constriction of scores on the digit-span test has acted to lower the correlation between the two tests. You decide to do the study again, this time using a much broader sample.

You go to the beach and ask every person you walk up to if he or she will participate in your new study. You give both tests to the first 30 people who agree to participate, and you collect information about their ages and levels of education that confirms that this subject group is much less homogeneous than the college group. This time, the correlation between your test and the digit-span test is .42, a statistically significant correlation. You now have a study that can be used to provide support for the construct validity of your inventory.

You've learned something from your first validity study about the impact sampling can have on research findings. As you begin the process of trying to validate the relationship between focus and actual performance, you have an important choice to make. How broad a subject sample do you want? Do you think your hypothesis applies equally well to all sports? Do you think it applies equally well to males and to females? How about the age of the athlete and the level of experience; will these things make a difference? What about cultural factors? Is it conceivable that in general, members of some cultures are more focused than are members of other cultures?

Any differences that do exist as a function of type of sport, age, sex, experience, etc., will increase the variability in test scores and will increase the correlation that you find. If you restrict yourself to testing highly homogeneous groups like world-class divers, for example, will there be enough variability in subject scores on your measure and on any measure of performance for you to obtain a decent-sized correlation? Then, too, will you be able to generalize your results to other, less homogeneous groups?

You decide to conduct your first test on college football players. It's a strategic decision for several reasons. First, you have access to a large number of them. Second, you don't expect the range of scores for a group of college football players to be as constricted as the range of some other athlete groups might be. Third, if you intend to market your instrument in the future, there are a lot of people playing football, and football programs have the money to pay for testing.

You go to the football coach and ask him how skills and overall performance are evaluated. Ultimately, you come up with a rating scale the coach uses to evaluate each player along two dimensions. The coach gives each athlete a score ranging from 1 to 100 on the basis of the athlete's (a) dedication and focus and (b) overall performance.

You administer your inventory to the 60 players trying out for the team and collect the coach's ratings. You then correlate both ratings with the players' scores on your inventory. The correlation between the coach's ratings of dedication and focus and the athletes' scores on your test is .52. The correlation between the coach's ratings of performance and your inventory is .40. With 60 subjects in your study, you need a correlation of .25 for the results to be statistically significant. You conclude that your measure of focus is related to the performance of college football players. Your study has added to the validity of your instrument.

How Useful Is the Inventory?

You now have an instrument with some internal consistency, reliability, and validity. It measures an individual's focus and dedication, and it has been shown to be significantly related to performance. How useful is this measure? If you were working with a football team and were qualified to use and interpret the inventory, would you use it?

The first question you should ask yourself is "Will the inventory help me find out anything about performance that I wouldn't find out quickly enough anyway?" Forget for the moment issues of validity and reliability. To be useful, the information you obtain from the inventory must add to your knowledge in a significant way. If there is reason to believe it will improve your ability to predict performance, and this is important, then you might consider using it. If there is reason to believe it will enhance your ability to anticipate and to prevent problems, and this is important, you might consider using it. If there is reason to believe it will help you accelerate the learning process, for example, by helping a player adjust to the team or to a new coach, then you might want to use it.

Looking at this inventory on focus, do you think it has the potential to help you in any of these ways? The answer is no, for the following reasons:

- The characteristic of focus measured by the inventory is easily observable in the athlete's behavior. You see it in the athlete's attitude and behavior during practice. You see it in the people with whom the athlete chooses to associate. You see it in how the athlete spends his or her spare time.

- Coaches are especially sensitive to how dedicated and focused their players are. The inventory does not present the athlete or the coach with a performance-relevant variable of which they are not already aware. The instrument does not help them to look at the variable in a new way. The coach will not overlook the relevance of focus to performance, and the test isn't likely to provide information that the coach won't quickly become aware of on his or her own.

- The fact that the inventory measures only focus and dedication contributes to its lack of utility. Without examining the athlete's level of focus and dedication within the context of other personality characteristics, or "building blocks," of performance, you will not know how to control or to modify the athlete's level of focus and intensity. How do you use a high score or a low score? Even the most focused athletes have times when they lose their focus; likewise, the most unfocused athletes have times when they focus very well. What determines the conditions under which the athlete will focus? If the test told you that, it would be useful to you, to the athlete, and to the coach.

- We will discuss the predictive utility of the measure in more detail later, but the fact that the measure of focus correlates .40 with the coach's ratings of performance is not overly impressive. The athlete's ability to focus is only accounting for 16% of the variance in his performance. Obviously there are many other factors that play a more substantial role (e.g., talent). Because focus accounts for so little, never blindly use the measure to make a selection decision. (You should never use any inventory in this way, no matter how high the correlation.)

Let's assume that you expand your test. You develop additional scales that provide information about the conditions under which the athlete will and will not focus effectively. You obtain similar reliability and validity coefficients for the new scales that you add to your inventory. Then, you approach me and ask me if I am interested in using the test.

As I read the information you have provided, I come across a statement telling me that you can help me to identify the conditions under which an athlete will and will not focus effectively. From my experience as a coach, I know that it often takes me months, if not years, to find this out about most of my athletes. The reason it takes so long is simple.

With athletes who are extremely unfocused, everything seems to interfere. These individuals don't survive long in highly competitive environments. With athletes who are extremely focused, the times they fail to focus are few and far between. Even with the average athlete, the coach will have to observe behavior over a fairly long period of time before he or she will be able to identify, with any consistency, the conditions that seem to be contributing to the athlete's success and failure. Additionally, to find these consistencies, the coach must have both the analytical skills and the external awareness required to make those observations and connections. He or she must also have the time and the opportunity. How many athletes is the coach concerned about at one time? The more athletes the coach has, the more complicated the process will be and the longer it will take to identify the conditions that contribute to an individual's ability to focus.

If your inventory can help me to more quickly identify the conditions under which athletes are able to remain focused and disciplined, I'll use it. I'm interested—now I need to look at the evidence you have pulled together to show me that the inventory has a chance of doing what you are telling me it will do.

Interpreting Reliability and Validity Coefficients

You know that psychological inventories must be reliable and valid, but how do you know whether the validity and reliability coefficients, or correlations, that are reported for the inventory are high enough? Fortunately, there are some general guidelines you can use.

Correlations Between Items and the Total Score of the Test or Scale to Which They Contribute

Any correlation reported as supportive of the reliability or validity of an inventory should be statistically significant. On the other hand, as we have pointed out, it is possible for correlations to be highly significant and yet to account for very little of the variability in scores. It is also possible for a correlation to account for a very large percentage of the variability in scores and still be nonsignificant. The size of the correlation required for statistical significance depends on the number of subjects in the study; the more subjects, the smaller the correlation needed.

If the correlation between an item and the total score is extremely high (e.g., above .90), you should question whether or not you need all of the items in the scale or test. For example, if you construct a 10-item test and 1 of those items correlates 1.0 with the total score, then that item alone would give you the same information you would get when you administered all 10 items.

Some researchers have argued that correlations between the items on a scale and the total score should be moderately high (e.g., .50 to .80). This is not necessarily so. Ideally, you want to develop a scale that will be useful for making critical and subtle distinctions among people at the more extreme ends of your sample. It is the lesser-correlated items that can help you do that. Items that are statistically significant and fall between .30 and .80 are acceptable.

How High Should Test-Retest Reliability Coefficients Be?

When you are trying to evaluate test-retest reliability coefficients, you must be sensitive to the time elapsed between testing and retesting. It should be obvious that the longer the time interval between test administrations, the greater the opportunity for change; thus, you would expect test-retest reliability coefficients to decrease over time.

From a test-development standpoint, what is a reasonable interval between tests? If you look at the literature, you will see that most investigators provide test-retest reliability coefficients over intervals ranging from 1 or 2 weeks to a year. Most psychological inventories report 2-week test-retest reliability coefficients that range from around .60 to .90. One-year test-retest coefficients are slightly lower, ranging from .50 to .80.

These are some benchmarks you can use, but keep the following in mind. The content measured by the scale or test will have a significant effect on the test-retest reliability coefficient. If you ask questions related to emotions and moods (with answers such as "I feel ashamed"), you can expect lower test-retest reliability coefficients. Moods change often. If the inventory asks questions that have a factual and presumably unchanging answers (e.g., "I competed in sports in high school"), the test-retest correlations should be much higher.

Evaluating Construct and Concurrent Validity Coefficients

In the example presented earlier, we correlated the measure of focus with a subtest on another inventory that was also presumed to measure one aspect of focus. Our correlation was significant, but was it high enough? Did it account for as much of the variance as we would have hoped? If you came to us with your test and told us that it correlated .90 or higher with another measure of the same construct, why would we want to use it instead of the other inventory—an inventory that would have undoubtedly been in existence longer than yours? The correlation between the two would be so high that they could be giving us the same information. Under these conditions, I would make my choice based on considerations such as which people have used both instruments in the past (e.g., which one do the people I know use?), the ease of administration, and the cost.

When you consider correlations between similar measures of the same construct, you must determine how similar the definitions of the construct are. "Focus" on the digit-span subtest, for example, is limited to a very narrow type of focus that lasts for only a few seconds at a time. This is only one aspect of the focus and dedication we were trying to measure, so we would not expect a very high correlation. Indeed, if the correlation between the two was extremely high, we would wonder whether our broader measure was measuring dedication and long-term focus at all.

Evidence of concurrent validity is provided by any significant correlation between one measure of a construct and another measure of that same construct. It is also provided by any significant correlation between your measure of the construct and the behavior that you would predict based on the construct (e.g., a correlation between your measure of focus and the amount of time the athlete spends in practice).

Evaluating the Predictive Validity of Tests

Assume that you have conducted several studies, and all of them show a significant relationship between your measure of focus and athletes' performance. Regardless of whether you test athletes before they begin competing and then correlate their scores on your inventory with performance ratings made at the end of the season, or test them and rate their performance at the end of the season, the results are always the same. There is always a significant correlation between your inventory and the athletes' performance.

Now, assume that the correlation between your inventory and performance for athletes competing in the sport of diving is a perfect 1.0. Simply by administering your test at the start of the season, you can predict the overall performance of every diver on the team. You can now rank-order them, from first to last. Would the inventory be useful as a selection tool? Clearly it would. If the coach had to cut some divers from the team, the inventory would ensure that he cut the worst performers. Under these conditions, however, the inventory would probably not be useful as a training tool. First, correlations between two events, in this case your inventory and the athletes' diving performance, mean that there is a relationship. It does not necessarily mean that there is a *causal* relationship. The correlation has not excluded the presence of a causal relationship, but your research certainly has not established such; to demonstrate a causal relationship, you would have to show that changes in one variable always affect the other.

The second reason to doubt that your inventory would be useful as a training tool is that the correlation is perfect. Because you are testing the divers at the beginning of the year, and the performance ratings come at the end of the year, any change in one athlete's level of performance must be being mirrored perfectly by changes in the other athletes' levels of performance. Either that, or more likely, no one's performance is changing, and no learning is taking place.

This brings up a very important point. Is it reasonable to expect or to hope for perfect correlations when you are trying to predict performance? Upon reflection, your answer should be NO! Here are some of the reasons you should not expect perfect correlations, or even extremely high correlations, when you are predicting performance:

- Athletes who train and compete for an entire season will almost certainly improve their level of performance, and the degree of improvement is likely to differ from athlete to athlete.

- Talent and focus make a difference. There are athletes who are physically more gifted than others. What they lose in focus, they make up for with pure talent.

- Some athletes will sustain injuries, and their performance will suffer as a result. Had they been able to practice and to compete consistently, they would have had a better performance rating at the end of the year.

- Some athletes will have motivational and emotional problems that will interfere with their ability to perform during the year.

- Some athletes will exaggerate and minimize their abilities when responding to your inventory.

- In sports that are evaluated subjectively (e.g., diving), there will be athletes who are judged unfairly during the competition and end up being rated lower than they should have been.

- There will be some athletes for whom an act of fate or chance interfered to cause them to perform better or worse than they might have otherwise.

These are just some of the reasons you will not obtain, and should not expect, perfect correlations between your measure and athletes' performance. Perfect correlations leave no room for intervention. If you hope to make a living as a service provider, you will have to demonstrate that people's performance can change as a result of your interventions. The higher the correlation between your measure and athletes' performance, the less room there is for change.

How High Should Your Correlation (Validity Coefficient) Be?

How closely should a measure you develop to predict performance correlate with performance? Unfortunately, there is no simple answer to this question. Two factors can strongly influence how your measure will correlate with performance. The first relates to the characteristic you are measuring. How stable is it over time, and how great a role does it play in performance? If your predictor variable is speed in the 100-meter races (at the beginning of track season), and performance is based on the athlete's finish in 100-meter races over the season, you will probably have a higher correlation than if your predictor variable is focus of attention. This is especially true when the physical skill levels (or talent) of the athletes in the sample are highly variable. It is less true when the variability in the physical skills of the athlete (e.g., speed) is smaller.

The second factor that will influence the correlation is the extent to which you can control things like injuries, false starts, and disqualifications. Response bias, accidents, and emotional problems will affect the correlation. This is one reason that, independent of how high predictive correlations should be, most of those presented in the literature fall between .30 and .40 and account for 10% to 15% of the variance.

Of What Relevance Are the Predictive Validity Studies of an Inventory?

Predictive validity allows you to generalize from your results. This may come as a surprise to you, but we are going to argue that the vast majority of predictive validity studies of inventories have no generalizability to diverse performance arenas. They can be used to provide support for the construct validity of the inventory, but it is risky to assume that the predictive power found in the reported studies can be directly applied to your assessment setting or situation.

Anyone attempting to use the GRE, for example, to help predict the performance of females in graduate school would find that despite the test's apparent overall predictive validity for graduate students, it does not hold for women (Sternberg & Williams, 1997). There are just too many differences between subjects and between competitive environments, no matter how closely related the groups appear to be.

The Normal Distribution

Of the theoretical assumptions that underlie the use of correlation coefficients, one is critical, namely, the assumption that the kind of characteristics under examination are "normally distributed" throughout the general population. To illustrate our point, let's go back to our study correlating a college coach's performance ratings with athlete focus. Figure 11 shows what a normal distribution looks like for the measure of focus we created for football players. When we administered the measure of focus to the college football team, the average (or mean) score was 30, and the standard deviation was 5.

As you can see from Figure 11, 68% of the players tested had focus scores that ranged between 25 and 35. Only 3% of the athletes had focus scores at or above 45, and only another 3% of them had scores at or below 20.

Statisticians and psychologists assume that any human characteristic or behavior will be normally distributed across the population being evaluated. Thus, a graph identical to the one shown in Figure 11 could be created to show how the coach's performance ratings were distributed across the population.

Let's say that the mean performance rating the coach assigned to players was 70 and that the standard deviation was 10. This means that 68% of the players had performance ratings that fell between 60 and 80. Three percent of the players had performance ratings of 80 or higher, and 3% of the players had performance ratings of 50 or lower.

Now you compute the correlation between the coach's rating of performance and the athlete's self-rating of focus. The correlation you obtain is .40, which is statistically significant. You have established some validity for your inventory, but do you think that the relationship between your measure of focus and the coach's rating of player performance will be as strong for a group of professional football players?

What would you anticipate would happen to the two distributions of scores if you were to examine professional players rather than college players? It is conceivable that the mean performance rating assigned by the coach and the variability in the ratings assigned by the coach would remain the same. The ratio of great players and poor players on a team won't

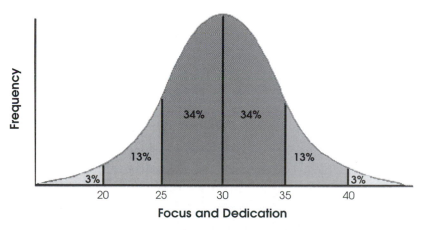

Figure 11. The normal distribution.

change when you are evaluating the individuals in relation to their peers. Of the players in college, 3% will be stars, and the same percentage will be stars in the pro ranks. In both cases, 3% percent will wash out. There is no reason, however, to assume that the measure of focus and dedication will remain the same across the two groups. College athletes have to split their focus between their sport and academics; pros do not. We would expect professional athletes to be more focused and dedicated. We would expect their mean scores on the measure of focus to be higher and the amount of variability to be less. We look at their scores and find this to be the case. The mean score for focus is 40 for pros, and the standard deviation is 2.5. This means that 68% of the pros scored between 37.5 and 42.5 on the focus inventory.

Under these circumstances, the correlation between focus and performance may be weakened because of the changes in the distributions. The opposite might also occur. You might find that at the professional level, focus becomes more important as a predictor and that the correlation increases because the level of talent across athletes is more consistent than it is in college competition. You are more likely to find this, however, if the distribution of scores is not too constricted.

The point we are trying to make is that you must be careful how you interpret and use the information you read about the predictive validity of an inventory. At best, the fact that an inventory shows some predictive power in relationship to a particular group suggests that it might provide you with similar information.

The information we have just given you about the predictive power of psychological tests should make it very clear why tests should never be used in isolation to make important decisions— selection decisions, for example. It should also be clear that predictive validity studies do more to establish the construct validity than the predictive power of psychological instruments. There is no substitute for critical common sense or evaluating statistical concepts and techniques.

When and How You Should Use Psychological Tests

Of course we aren't suggesting that tests aren't useful or that they can't be used for selection. As we have stated before, we believe just the opposite. Because there are very real limitations to the predictive power of psychological inventories, however, people often must revise their expectations about what they can learn from tests and how they can use them.

Here are the key questions we would raise before using a psychological test:

- Is the inventory reliable?

- Does it measure the constructs it claims to measure, and are those constructs directly related to making relevant decisions?

- Does it promise to provide information that can add significantly to the speed of decision making or to the accuracy of important decisions— decisions about selection, placement, training, or the integration of an individual into a program?

- Is it cost-effective? In other words, is the information gained worth the price?

Notice that we have not indicated a specific concern with predictive validity. Predictive validity is best understood as a type of construct validity. If you look at the predictive validity studies that have been conducted on virtually any psychological inventory you choose, you will find that very few of them can be generalized to any of the subject populations you would test. The unavoidable fact is that you will probably have to establish the predictive validity of your entire assessment process every time you engage in it. You must consider predictive validity in the context of the entire assessment process, especially in your need for intervention-relevant information. Here, the emphasis is on getting information you can use, not just information that meets some abstract, artificial, statistical standard.

Probabilities and Tendencies Versus Absolutes

You want to use test information to make predictions about people's behavior. You then want to use these predictions to help you make important decisions. Should you select the athlete for the team? Will he or she perform better as a team leader or as a role player? How can you improve his or her performance under pressure? What steps can you take to help an athlete get along with the other members of the team?

The right tests—those that meet the criteria we have just identified—can help you make predictions or testable hypotheses more quickly than you would otherwise. The right tests can provide information that will help you to determine the specific steps you must take to change behavior and to improve performance. (No test, however, can make any predictions with the degree of accuracy required to allow decisions to be made by tests rather than by people.)

Statistically significant tests provide information that allows you to make predictions about *response tendencies*. Response tendencies can have an important influence on the ultimate success of the individual and the team. Tests can also provide information that will help you to determine the conditions that are more or less likely to increase the frequency of certain responses. Because these predicted tendencies are less than perfect, it is your job to attempt to find additional confirmatory evidence of the tendencies and their usefulness. This is consensual validation, the process we discussed in chapter 3.

The assessment process, whether you employ tests or not, ends only when you have collected enough information to make the most responsible decision possible. This decision must be one that will withstand the careful examination of a jury of your peers. Of course, the more critical the decision, the more careful you have to be in your practice.

Ultimately, you will use tests to provide structure and to help ensure that attention is paid to the broad range of human characteristics that have direct implications for performance. You will also use tests as early warning systems, to sensitize you to possible problems. Always gather additional information to provide assurance that the issues identified by an inventory are indeed real and are relevant to the decisions you make.

Suggested Readings

Eyde, L. D., Robertson, G. J., Krug, S. E., Moreland, K. L., Robertson, A. G., Shewan, C. M., Harrison, P. L., Porch, B. E., Hammer, A. L., & Primoff, E. S., (1993). *Responsible test use: Case studies for assessing human behavior.* Washington, DC: American Psychological Association.

Schutz, R. W., & Gessaroli, M. E. (1993). Use, misuse, and disuse of psychometrics in sport psychology research. In R. N. Singer, M. Murphey, & L. K. Tennant (Eds.), *Handbook of research on sport psychology* (pp. 901–917). New York: Macmillan.

Sternberg, R. J., & Williams, W. M. (1997). Does the Graduate Record Examination predict meaningful success in the graduate training of psychologists? A case study. *American Psychologist, 52*(6), 630–641.

Reading and Evaluating the Research Literature

11

In chapter 10, we provided a very basic description of correlations and how they are used. You should now be able to understand the arguments presented in this chapter. Over the years, we have noticed that the research literature within sport psychology has not been very supportive of assessment. There are many reasons for this, and in this chapter we will discuss the two that we believe are most important.

Inventories Appropriate for Sport Psychology

The first reason the literature has not been favorable is that many of the tests that have been used in sport were designed for clinical use and have been inappropriately applied within the sport psychology arena. To us, some of this criticism is justified. The use of instruments such as the Minnesota Multiphasic Personality Inventory and the Rorschach with athlete populations is extremely difficult to justify. The constructs measured by these instruments have no direct relationship to performance (Kubie, 1952).

Projective techniques like the Rorschach were designed to help clinicians understand abnormal and irrational behavior. They are based on psychoanalytic theories that have done little to improve our ability to predict and to control behavior. The Minnesota Multiphasic Personality Inventory was developed statistically, without a preconceived theoretical basis, to identify the characteristics associated with the psychiatric labels applied to patients. Its primary use is as a diagnostic tool to help professionals assign labels to patients with serious psychological problems (Hathaway & McKinley, 1940, 1943; Meehl, 1954).

The incidence of clinical problems is no greater in sport than in the general population. For the most part, sport psychologists are working with healthy individuals. Because this is the case, the behaviors these individuals engage in, even when they "fall apart under pressure," can be explained without resorting to psychodynamic theories postulating underlying pathology. We do take issue with the conclusion of many researchers that sport-specific measures are more useful and valid than more general measures. For these researchers, it isn't enough that instruments are performance-relevant; they must be sport-relevant or even specific-sport relevant (Ebbeck, 1991). Let's look at a couple of the assumptions that underlie this position and then compare these assumptions with the reasons for testing.

Sport-Specific Measures Versus General Measures

The primary assumption underlying the use of sport-specific measures is that behavior is principally situation-specific. We would argue, however, that personality characteristics, attitudes, and values that are especially entrenched become traitlike as pressure increases within the performance situation. The more traitlike characteristics become for an athlete, the more predictive they are of behavior across situations.

Another assumption, although probably an implicit one for most researchers, is that the primary goal of assessment is the prediction of behavior. However, it is possible to predict behavior without having any understanding of the factors that contribute to that behavior. For example, a fan doesn't have to know anything about a sport to know which team has the best record. If that fan consistently supports the team with the best record, he or she will do a better job of predicting performance than will the person who does not. The job of a sport psychologist, however, isn't merely to predict behavior. In fact, any good coach will predict overall behavior more effectively than will a sport psychologist, because the coach will be more skilled at evaluating the relative technical and tactical strengths of the athletes or teams. The sport psychologist will help the coach make more accurate predictions by helping him or her understand the psychological variables that affect behavior when technical and tactical talent alone doesn't provide an explanation. We will argue that the sport psychologist's efforts to provide information to the coach will be more effective if the psychologist does not limit assessment to a sport-specific situation. Figure 12 shows the differences that can occur in a subject's responses to TAIS when the subject is given a sport-specific response set.

Figure 12 shows our world-champion gymnast's scores on TAIS under two different response-set conditions. The first response set was very general. Ludmilla was told that the inventory measured concentration and interpersonal skills important for performance. She was also told that information from the inventory would be used to help her improve her concentration skills. Immediately after she responded to the inventory, we asked Ludmilla if

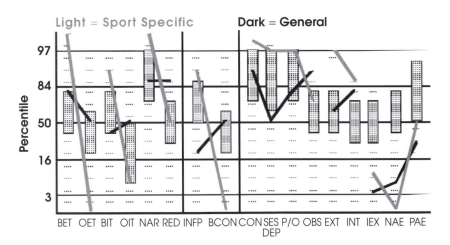

Figure 12. Gymnast's TAIS scores, sport-specific vs. general response set.

she would answer the questions a second time to help us with our research. This time, she was told to read each item and to relate it specifically to her sport. In other words, she was to mentally translate the items on TAIS to make them sport-specific. She was also told that the average gymnast against whom she competed would answer "sometimes" to most of the items on the inventory. When responding, Ludmilla was to compare herself with her average competitor. Ludmilla's scores under the second response set are shown as lighter lines.

If we were interested in using Ludmilla's scores on TAIS to predict whether or not she would make the Olympic team, we would have been more accurate had we given her a sport-specific response set. Looking at Ludmilla's scores, you might be tempted to draw the conclusion that a sport-specific response set, especially when combined with instructions designed to make sure she compared herself with an appropriate comparison group (e.g., Olympic-level competitors, in this case), is the way to go. Before drawing this conclusion, however, ask yourself these questions:

- Why am I testing the athlete?

- What do I want to learn about the athlete?

Predicting Performance for Purposes of Selection

Let's assume you want to use your inventory to select members of the Olympic team. Based on Ludmilla's scores, you might think that giving sport-specific measures and controlling the athlete's choice of a comparison group are good ideas, but how likely do you think the average athlete would be to exaggerate his or her scores if he or she thought the inventory was being used for selection? In a selection situation, the more face validity your inventory has, the easier it is to exaggerate or fake. There is little doubt that a performance-relevant measure that has good face validity, when administered under a response set that forces the athlete to compare him- or herself with the competition, should have greater predictive power than a more general questionnaire. Whether the sport-specific measure will be more predictive, however, will depend on the athlete's level of honesty and cooperation.

Even if an athlete cooperates, what have you learned? The best predictor of performance is past behavior. A good coach will be better able to tell you who is going to make the team than will your sport-specific inventory. It's doubtful that the specific response set will significantly improve your prediction of performance; indeed, it's much more likely that providing a specific response set will prevent the athlete from telling you things about him- or herself that would allow you to be of help. The specific response set is apt to mask issues that influence her ability to perform; with it, you often obtain less information than you need.

Predicting the Conditions That Influence Performance

What do you want to learn about the athlete? If you want to learn about the conditions that lead to the ups and downs in his or her performance, then you don't want to impose so much structure on the athlete's responses that you prevent him or her from providing that information.

When we work with athletes, how they are performing is important. Perhaps even more important is how they are feeling about themselves and about their performance—not just in their sport, but in other aspects of their lives as well. Even focused athletes are people, and they are not immune to what goes on outside the competitive arena. For instance, relationships with significant others have an impact on performance, if not immediately, then certainly in the long run.

Neither the coach nor Ludmilla needed a psychological inventory to know that Ludmilla would make the Olympic team and would perform well in competition. The coach wasn't interested in predicting Ludmilla's performance; he wanted intervention-relevant information. Ludmilla's responses under the more general response set indicated that she was not particularly interested in telling us about her actual performance. She wanted to tell us how she was feeling. It was an appreciation of her feelings that would help the coach to understand her better.

How do you explain breakdowns in performance when athletes have the physical talent and the technical and tactical knowledge required to perform, but fail to do so? Isn't this what sport psychologists are trying to predict, understand, and control? If it is, then it is important that we assess more than the level at which the athlete is currently competing. We need to observe how the athlete's self-concept affects his or her behavior. We need to know what the athlete thinks and feels about his or her performance, and we must gain insight into the impact that the larger environment (e.g., relationships to family, friends, country) has on the individual. Knowledge about the athlete's performance provides the benchmark we use to begin evaluating the athlete's cognitive and emotional characteristics. Effective coaching and performance enhancement require information from each of these areas.

Problems in the Research Literature

Another reason the research literature has been skeptical about testing involves test validation and outcome research. Poor design and unrealistic assumptions have, not surprisingly, led to negative findings (Martens, 1975; Morgan, 1980; Silva, 1984). Here are a few examples:

- Studies are designed with the implicit assumption that there is a linear relationship between the predictor variable, whatever that may be, and performance. The higher the score on the predictor variable, the better the performance. This implicit assumption is often incorrect. For example, athletes can have performance problems because they are too competitive. To make the simple assumption that a high competitive score is good and a low one is bad is simplistic.

- Many researchers fail to account for, or to control, subject response sets. They administer tests for research purposes at a selection camp for the Olympic games, for example, and fail to take into account the situational factors that will influence responses to the inventories. The lack of trust in many research situations leads subjects to exaggerate strengths and to minimize weaknesses.

- Researchers design studies to predict the outcome of particular events rather than to examine response tendencies and performance over time. Psychological test scores indicate behavioral tendencies. For example, a high score on the external distractibility scale on TAIS suggests that the person has a tendency to become distracted. You are more likely to validate that scale by observing behavior over time than by observing behavior in one isolated situation.

- Researchers design studies that fail to consider the importance of mediating variables like arousal. For example, they predict performance differences between groups based on such factors as external awareness. In the process, they ignore an underlying theoretical postulate that concentration differences will develop only when arousal levels increase to the point of interfering with the individual's ability to shift focus of attention.

- Researchers evaluate theories incorrectly because of the perceived need for statistical independence among predictor variables (Nideffer, 1987).

Researchers are often guilty of treating predictor variables as pure traits and of exhibiting insensitivity to the complexities of human behavior (Fisher, 1984).

The State-Trait Issue

For years there have been arguments in the literature about the relative permanence of human characteristics. On an intellectual level, psychology has moved away from the pure state-trait dichotomy. Clearly, there are individuals who have certain characteristics they display independent of the situation. Their behavior is very predictable across situations and is therefore very traitlike (e.g., the person who can't seem to stop talking; the highly analytical individual who loses all awareness of the surroundings; and the individual who can't stop competing, even in social situations). We also see people who are able to adapt their behaviors quite easily to new situations. They can be like chameleons, blending into almost any background.

Increasing arousal typically causes highly developed cognitive and personality characteristics to become more traitlike and, thus, more predictive of the individual's behavior. Practitioners and researchers need to keep this in mind, especially when dealing with healthy populations. Healthy individuals tend to behave in more flexible or situation-specific ways than do individuals belonging to clinical populations. The ability to adapt appropriately to new situations is one of the definitions of healthy functioning. Healthy individuals tend to perform well over time and across situations precisely because they can make adjustments. Let's use TAIS data to illustrate the points we want to make here. The TAIS profile shown in Figure 13 is that of the average world champion.

Look at the attentional scales on the world-champion profile. The NAR scale, as you know, measures the athlete's ability to focus concentration, to pay attention to details, and to follow through. This scale is the highest attentional scale score and is the concentration skill we would expect to become increasingly traitlike as arousal increases. The OIT scale, which measures an individual's tendency to overanalyze and to overthink, is the lowest

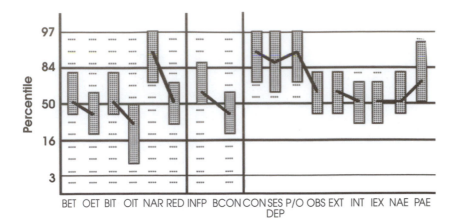

Figure 13. World-champion profile.

scale score on the concentration side of the profile. You do not normally think of distractibility as a skill or a habit, but if you do, you'll realize that as pressure increases, the world champion is least likely to overanalyze. If anything, he or she will become too focused and inflexible.

With respect to the state-trait issue, you should interpret the concentration, intrapersonal, and interpersonal characteristics of normal and supernormal individuals in the following way: Forget about the absolute elevation of scores when you are looking at the profile of an individual as opposed to a group profile like the one shown in Figure 13. Individual profiles are subject to response-set and response-style influences that can inappropriately raise and lower scores relative to the mean for the group. These influences tend to cancel each other out in a group profile.

Draw two lines across the profile, like the lighter ones shown in Figure 14. The first line should represent the mean for all six concentration scores. The second line should represent the mean for the interpersonal scales. The scores near the mean are least likely to become increasingly traitlike as pressure builds.

The athlete's profile in Figure 14 is quite similar to the average-world-record-holder profile, just a little more extreme, possibly due to a different response set or response style. Drawing lines across the profile to define the average attentional and interpersonal score for the individual helps you to identify which specific behaviors will increase and become more traitlike (scores way above the line) and which will decrease across situations (scores way below the line) as pressure increases.

Under a normal amount of pressure, the average world-record holder will not make many mistakes. He or she will perform well, even in situations that require analytical thinking, most likely the athlete's least developed attentional skill. It is only as pressure begins to increase that the athlete loses flexibility and relies more heavily on preferred or more highly developed behavior. Under pressure, our world-record holder becomes more focused (NAR), less distractible (OET, OIT), more controlling (CON), more self-confident, less willing to listen (SES), more competitive (P/O), more positive (PAE), and less verbal (IEX). These are great characteristics for most high-level competitive situations, but such characteristics may not be so positive if they emerge in another performance arena—an arena in which the athlete is under

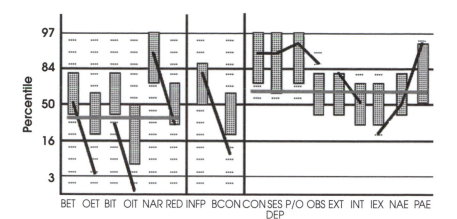

Figure 14. Finding the subject's mean score.

pressure and is required to be flexibile, cooperative, and attentive to what others say.

Researchers attempting to predict the performance of healthy individuals, particularly individuals with the same technical and tactical skills and knowledge, must manipulate arousal levels. Practitioners must keep in mind that it does not work to simply classify subjects according to their dominant concentration styles and expect to find differences in behavior without systematically manipulating emotional arousal. Just because profile differences indicate that an individual's more dominant or traitlike characteristics are not ideally suited to the performance arena (e.g., a world champion is dominated by an analytical focus of concentration instead of a narrow focus), this does not mean that the athlete will fail or that problems are inevitable. It is essential to assess the athlete's ability to control arousal and emotion. If the performance arena doesn't generate enough emotional arousal to cause the athlete to lose flexibility, he or she will perform well. Implicit here is the view that athletes have to perform under pressure. If the arousal level is not sufficiently high, you may never discover important psychological strengths and weaknesses.

The Role of the Overload Scales on TAIS

The world-champion shooter profiled in Figure 15 is experiencing a temporary crisis. As a result, he is more emotional and more easily loses control over emotions and focus. His tendencies to become distracted (OET), overloaded (OIT), and unable to make appropriate shifts in focus of concentration (RED) have all become more traitlike.

With TAIS, you can use scores on the distractibility (OET), overload (OIT), reduced-focus (RED), and speed-of-decision-making (OBS) scales to gauge the relative ease with which individuals will lose control over their emotions and their ability to concentrate and perform.

Remember that in Figure 15, you are dealing with a world-record holder. His scores are not so high that you would expect him to be unable to perform. Because he is involved in a closed-skill sport, one that allows him to determine when to pull the trigger, he should be able to wait until he has cleared out the distractions and is ready to perform.

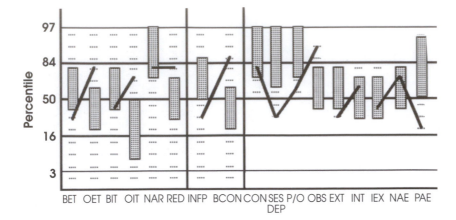

Figure 15. When distractibility and the inability to shift become traitlike.

Statistical Dependence and Independence

Another important problem concerns the concept of statistical independence (Schultz & Gessaroli, 1993). Incorrect assumptions about the need for psychological characteristics to be statistically independent of one another often cause both researchers and the individuals evaluating the research literature to draw inappropriate conclusions about the validity of tests. These mistakes are most often seen in

- studies that have been designed to replicate earlier studies (e.g., studies attempting to replicate the factor structure of an inventory or a regression equation that has been used to predict performance); and

- factor-analytic studies in which the researcher is attempting to use the factor structure of the inventory to confirm the independent existence of the different constructs measured by the inventory.

As you read the next few paragraphs, try to keep in mind the basic information we presented about correlation coefficients and the amount of variance for which they account. If you do, you will begin to realize that having or establishing statistical independence between different psychological characteristics should not be considered a goal for test developers or an ideal for practitioners.

In chapter 10, we stated that a correlation coefficient measures the interdependence of two variables. If the correlation between the two variables is 0.0, we assume that the variables are completely independent of one another. If we test 100 subjects and obtain a correlation of .20, we know that the two variables are dependent upon each other in a statistically significant way. The amount of variance accounted for, however, is only 4%.

While it is true that in this example the variables show some dependence, they actually show more independence. In fact, 96% of the variability between the two sets of scores remains to be explained. The same is true with a correlation coefficient of .71. A dependent relationship clearly exists between the two variables, yet 50% of the variance goes unexplained.

Researchers often confuse conceptual independence with statistical independence. We will use scales on TAIS to illustrate the difference. From a conceptual standpoint, the ability to focus one's attention externally (BET) can be thought of as independent of the ability to develop a broad-internal focus (BIT), which can be thought of as distinct from the ability to develop a very narrow focus of attention (NAR). Likewise, from a conceptual standpoint, we can separate an individual's willingness to take control (CON) from his level of self-confidence (SES) and his level of interpersonal competitiveness (P/O).

From a standpoint of overall performance, however, we should not expect these constructs to be completely statistically independent, or *orthogonal*. For example, solving problems effectively (BIT) requires an awareness of the environment (BET) because external information is often relevant to the problem. Problem solving also requires focused concentration to develop and implement solutions (NAR). Considering this, we would expect to see positive correlations among these three conceptually different concentration skills. They should not be completely independent.

The same is true on the interpersonal side of the profile. If individuals are confident (SES), they usually have reason to be so. Confident individuals are often confident because they are in control of situations (CON) and because they have good attentional skills (BET, BIT, NAR) and are not easily distracted (negative correlations with OET, OIT, RED). For these reasons, confident individuals are more likely to be competitive (P/O) and positive (PAE). Common sense tells us that these scales should be correlated and should not be statistically independent in any absolute sense.

Too often, researchers design validity studies as if the different characteristics measured by tests were completely independent. When they do, they look at variables (e.g., focus of concentration) in isolation, a perspective that dramatically oversimplifies the demands of most performance situations and fails to control for other, mediating variables.

To allow you to understand how unreasonable these expectations are, we will use an example that has nothing to do with psychology. Suppose you are a researcher and you want to predict performance in the 100 meters. You look at the athlete's body, and you generate some hypotheses about the physical attributes that contribute to performance. You know that the legs contribute, and you decide you can measure that contribution by measuring stride length and speed of turnover. You know that the arms contribute through their pumping action, and you find some way to measure that action. You know that hearing and sight contribute, to the extent that they allow the athlete to get a quick start, so you measure these variables. You collect a group of athletes whose performances in the 100 meters differ dramatically. Some are elite-level performers, some compete at the sub-elite level, and others run simply for fun.

You measure them on all these variables. Clearly, the variables discussed are conceptually independent. Arms are different from legs; stride length is different from speed of turnover, etc. When you look at the correlations between these variables, however, do you believe for one minute that they will be completely independent? Do you think that our measurement techniques are sophisticated enough to separate out the independent contribution of each of these variables? We might get some rough ideas, but common sense will tell you that there is enough interdependence between the variables that changes in one will be reflected in changes in others. Wholes do not comprise statistically independent parts. The athlete with the best combination of stride length and turnover would find both of these variables affected by the loss of the use of his or her arms.

If we did somehow manage to artificially and accurately separate out the independent contribution of each of these variables for the group tested, would we find the same relative contribution with another group? It's highly unlikely. In each group, there would be strengths in one area that acted to compensate for weaknesses in another. The result for both groups might be the same, but how they got there would be different. To understand how this confusion affects the literature, consider the use of *factor analysis* as a tool for developing and validating psychological inventories.

Using Factor Analysis

We administer TAIS to a large group of subjects, look at all of the subjects' scores, and find large differences among subjects in terms of their profile patterns and in terms of how high or low their scores are. We can refer to these collective differences in the scores as the amount of variability that exists among all of the subjects tested. Each subject taking TAIS is scored on 17 different scales (all of the things the test measures). Researchers use factor analysis to see if the scales are dependent upon each other (e.g., statistically correlated). If all 17 scales were completely independent, the correlations between the scales would be zero. The factor analysis would identify 17 factors (one for each scale), and each of these factors would account for approximately 6%, or 1/17, of the variance in the scores.

Given the arguments presented above, it is extremely unlikely that the scales would all correlate 0.0 with each other. In fact, we should have serious questions about what we are really measuring if they do. In real life, the variables we are trying to measure don't operate completely independently of each other. They are conceptually independent, but, in practice, they are significantly correlated with one another.

In the research literature, factor analytical solutions of most well-validated, multidimensional personality measures result in the identification of only five "independent" factors (Hogan, Hogan, & Roberts, 1996). These factors have been defined using a variety of terms, depending upon the researcher. Table 5 shows how they are seen on TAIS and what they seem to reflect.

The factors and the TAIS scales that load on the factors shown in Table 7 are reasonably constant across studies, but there is some variation depending upon the group tested. For example, in some studies, the conscientiousness factor consists of a high score on narrowing (NAR) and low scores on external distractibility (-OET), internal distractibility (-OIT), behavior control or impulsiveness (-BCON), and negative affect expression or confrontational attributes (-NAE). When that happens, the emotional stability factor consists of the subject's scores on internal distractibility (-OIT), reduced focus (-RED), and obsessiveness (-OBS). There are also times when the narrowing scale drops out of the factor reflecting conscientiousness, causing that factor to consist of the external distractibility scale (-OET), internal distractibility scale

Table 7. The Big Five Personality Factors

	TAIS scales
Intellectence—This dimension is associated with cognitive and analytical skills.	BET, BIT, INFP, IEX
Agreeableness—This dimension reflects extroversion and supportiveness.	EXT, PAE, -INT
Surgency—This dimension reflects leadership, confidence, and assertiveness.	CON, SES, P/O
Conscientiousness—This dimension reflects self-discipline and focus.	NAR
Emotional stability—This dimension is the opposite of anxious, worried, insecure, etc.	-OET, -OIT, -RED, -BCON, -NAE, OBS

(-OIT), behavior control scale (-BCON), and negative affect expression scale (-NAE).

Now why would you end up with five fairly consistent factors? Why would some TAIS scales, for instance, shift back and forth between factors or not load in a significant way on any factor? Most important, what are the implications of these changes? Do they mean that the inventory is invalid or unstable? We mentioned that factor analysis is a statistical program that looks at the test variables to see if they are related to one another. If they are, then the scales that are related represent *common profiles* of score patterns that are representative of many people, not just of one individual. These patterns account for much more of the total variance in test scores than does any single scale.

How the program actually works is somewhat complicated, but the essence of what it does is as follows: A *correlation matrix* is computed that correlates every scale on the inventory with every other scale. The program identifies some source of common variance across scales that correlate with one another. What we call that *common source of variance* depends on the individual scales that *load* (correlate) significantly with it. Every scale will correlate to one degree or another with the factor, but some will do so much more than others will. The first factor that gets separated out, depending on the type of factor analysis, will usually account for anywhere from 20% to 50% of the total variability in test scores. In other words, that factor will account for as much variability as anywhere from three to eight scales on TAIS, assuming the scales were all completely independent. Once that variance in scores has been explained, it is removed from further calculations. A second factor is then identified based on the remaining interscale correlations.

Here is an example to help clarify this. Let's say that there are correlations of .60 between analytical skill (BIT) and intellectual expressiveness (IEX), and the first factor (intellectance) that is extracted. This means that the first factor accounts for approximately 36% of the variance (the square of the .6 correlation) in both the BIT and IEX scores. Now, 64% of the variance of each scale remains to be accounted for; thus, each of these scales may still load significantly on factors yet to be extracted.

The second factor that is extracted will account for the next large portion of variability in scores. Let's say the second factor turns out to be the surgency, or leadership, factor. Again, all of the scales on the inventory will load on this factor, but some will load more heavily than others. The researchers who interpret the factor structures that evolve from the analysis employ a number of statistical strategies to help them with the process. After all, if every scale loads on every factor, things can get pretty confusing. In essence, the strategies the researchers use help them to isolate the scales that contribute most heavily to the factor. The flip side of this is that they ignore other scales that contribute to the factor. In practice, information gathered from these other scales might prove crucial. Obsession with the simplification afforded by factor analysis yields a cost in terms of information available to the practitioner (Cronbach, 1984; Hough, 1992).

Assume for argument's sake that our first factor accounts for 40% of the variance in scores and that our second factor, which consists primarily of the control scale (CON), the self-esteem scale (SES), and the physical orientation scale (P/O), accounts for another 25%. We now have two factors that account for as much of the variation in test scores as do 11 of the TAIS scales. Keep in mind here that the amount of variance accounted for by each factor reflects not only the variability attributed by the scales most strongly associated with the factor, but also the variability attributed by contributions made by all of the other scales. The process of extracting factors continues until the amount of variance accounted for by the last factor extracted drops below the amount of variance we would expect a single scale to contribute to the total variability in test scores. In the case of TAIS, because there are 17 scales contributing to the variability, when the amount of variance that is accounted for by a factor drops below 6% (or 1/17th of the total variability), the computer stops looking for factors. Researchers consider factors to be valid and reliable only if they account for more of the variance than a single scale would.

As you can see in the example provided, if the first two factors account for 65% of the variance (11 of the 17 TAIS scales), only 35% of the variability remains to be explained. This would allow, at most, the generation of 5 to 6 more factors. If this were the case, you would have an 8-factor solution instead of a 17-factor solution. A researcher who believes the factor structure of an inventory should mirror the different scales on the test would look at the 8 factors and insist that your test is not measuring 17 different characteristics; it is measuring only 8.

Why do most multidimensional personality inventories (those with between 15 and 25 scales) typically end up with five factors? It is because the variables they measure, though conceptually independent, are statistically related to one another. Also, the individuals who developed the inventories all happened to be interested in similar constructs. They were all interested in sociability of one kind or another; they were all interested in intelligence or cognitive processes in one way or another; they were all interested in leadership and dedication, and they were all interested in emotional stability.

Why would some scales shift back and forth between one factor and another, and why would some drop out entirely? Let's take the narrowing scale on TAIS as an example. The narrowing scale has a low to moderate correlation with all of the other scales. The first factor extracted is intellectance. NAR correlates with this factor, but not highly enough for it to be considered a primary contributor. The second factor extracted is surgency, or leadership. Again, NAR correlates and contributes in an important way to this factor (leaders must be able to focus), but not so strongly that it is identified as one of the primary variables. The same is true of Factor 3, which might be agreeableness.

At this point, the amount of variability remaining in the NAR scale is dramatically reduced. We have accounted for most of the variability of the NAR scale, but it has been left out of every factor. Depending on which factor is identified next (e.g., conscientiousness or emotional stability), NAR may or may not contribute enough to be identified as a primary contributor. At this level in the analysis, relatively small differences in the characteristics of different subject populations may make a difference in which scales load on a factor. With a group of world-record holders, for example, the variability of the group's scores on the narrowing scale (NAR) is much less than it is for the general population. This fact would cause the loading of NAR on the various factors to be different than it would be if the scores on the group tested were much more variable.

A researcher trying to replicate the attentional dimensions measured by TAIS might conduct a factor analysis and have the first factors that are identified explain so much of the variance that NAR fails to be identified as an independent factor and fails to load significantly enough on the other factors to be included in them. Based on this, the researcher would be likely to conclude that TAIS does not measure the narrowing of attention. Is the researcher right? Theoretically, he or she could be. It is conceivable that the narrowing scale doesn't correlate with anything because it is not really measuring anything. The items are such a mixture that they don't belong together at all. The problem is that the analysis used by the researcher does not prove that. All it does is show that the scale did not load highly enough to be included in the factor structure that was identified. Because performance-related constructs demonstrate statistical interdependence, and because factor-analytic solutions are stopped once the amount of variance accounted for drops below the amount attributed by a single scale, you can't use the analysis to conclude anything about the factors or scales that weren't identified. Instead, you must look elsewhere to validate or to invalidate the construct of narrowing. When you do that, there is ample evidence for the validity and reliability of the narrowing scale.

An analysis of the content of the narrowing scale (NAR) shows that the items have face validity; they do ask about focus of attention. Correlations among the individual items on the scale and the total scale score indicate the items are related. Test-retest data show that subjects' responses to the items are consistent over time. A comparison of the concentration strengths of different groups demonstrates construct validity for both the narrowing scale (NAR) and the scale measuring broad-internal awareness (BIT). World champions and engineers are highest on the narrowing scale; CEOs and upper-level executives are highest on the analytical scale (BIT). Distinguishing world-record holders on the basis of sex or ethnicity makes no difference; the ability to narrow and focus concentration is a hallmark of world champions, independent of their country of origin or their gender (Nideffer, Sagal, Lowry, & Bond, 2000).

Summary and Conclusions

Approach test manuals and the research literature with a healthy skepticism. Don't assume that anything published, even if it appears in a peer-reviewed journal, is correct. Problems with perspective exist everywhere; the research literature is no exception. As you read, ask yourself questions: Do the validity coefficients being reported fall within the range you might realistically expect? If they are unusually high or low, ask yourself why. Chances are you will find an answer by looking at the design of the study and at the way in which the researcher has defined the constructs he or she is measuring.

When you see test publishers and developers making claims for the predictive power of inventories, look carefully at the characteristics of the subjects whose behavior is being predicted. Ask yourself if there is any reason to believe that you would or would not have similar findings with your clients. Be cautious when reading the conclusions drawn by researchers. Are the conclusions justified by the data? This same point holds for trying to evaluate outcome studies. Quite often, the failure to obtain predicted findings is due to inappropriate hypotheses, to limitations in the design of the study, and to poorly conceived outcome measures.

Do the hypotheses generated by the researcher make sense in light of what you know about the very real complexities of performance situations? For example, does the analysis of data assume a linear relationship between predictor variables and outcome measure? If so, is that appropriate? As we pointed out, athletes who have very high scores on measures of self-confidence can fail to perform well, just as can athletes with very low scores. They typically fail for different reasons, however.

Finally, are the data reliable? What were the demands of the assessment situation? How would they have influenced the subjects' responses? Did the experimenter attempt to control for these?

Suggested Readings

Cronbach, L. J. (1984). *Essentials of psychological testing* (4th ed.). San Francisco: Harper & Row.

Duda, J. L. (1998). *Advances in sport and exercise psychology measurement*. Morgantown, WV: Fitness Information Technology, Inc.

Ebbeck, V. (199). The current practice of reporting psychometric properties in sport psychology research. In V. Ebbeck (Chair), *Questionnaire development in sport psychology research: Rejuvenating the psychometric process*. Symposium conducted at the meeting of the North American Society for the Psychology of Sport and Physical Activity, Asilomar, CA.

Fisher, A. C. (1984). New directions in sport personality research. In J. M. Silva & R. S. Weinberg (Eds.), *Psychological foundations of sport* (pp. 70–80). Champaign, IL: Human Kinetics.

Gauvin, L., & Russell, S. J. (1993). Sport-specific and culturally adapted measures in sport and exercise psychology research: Issues and strategies. In R. N. Singer, M. Murphey, & L. K. Tennant (Eds.), *Handbook of research on sport psychology* (pp. 891–900). New York: Macmillan.

Hathaway, S. R., & McKinley, J. C. (1940). A multiphasic personality schedule (Minnesota): I. Construction of the schedule. *Journal of Psychology, 10,* 249–254.

Hathaway, S. R., & McKinley, J. C. (1943). *Manual for administering and scoring the MMPI.* Minneapolis: University of Minnesota Press.

Hogan, R., Hogan, J., & Roberts, B. W. (1996). Personality measurement and employment decisions, questions and answers. *American Psychologist, 51,* 469–477.

Hough, L. M.(1992). The "Big Five" personality variables-construct confusion: Description versus prediction. *Human Performance, 5,* 139–155.

Kubie, L. S. (1952). Problems and techniques of psychoanalytic validation and progress. In E. Pumpian-Mindlin (Ed.), *Psychoanalysis as scienc.* Stanford, CA: Stanford University Press.

Martens, R. (1975). The paradigmatic crisis in American sport personology. *Sportwissenschaft, 5*: 9–24.

Meehl, P. E. (1954). *Clinical versus statistical prediction.* Minneapolis: University of Minnesota Press.

Morgan, W. P. (1980). The trait psychology controversy. *Research Quarterly for Exercise and Sport, 52,* 385–427.

Nideffer, R. M. (1987). Issues in the use of psychological tests in applied settings. *The Sport Psychologist, 1,* 18–28.

Schutz, R. W., & Gessaroli, M. E. (1993). Use, misuse, and disuse of psychometrics in sport psychology research. In R. N. Singer, M. Murphey, & L. K. Tennant (Eds.), *Handbook of research on sport psychology* (pp.901–917). New York: Macmillan.

Silva, J. M., III. (1984). Personality and sport performance: Controversy and challenge. In J. M. Silva & R. S. Weinberg (Eds.), *Psychological foundations of sport* (pp. 59–69). Champaign, IL: Human Kinetics.

Sternberg, R. J., & Williams, W. M. (1997). Does the Graduate Record Examination predict meaningful success in the graduate training of psychologists? A case study. *American Psychologist, 52*(6), 630–641.

The Future of Psychological Assessment in Sport

12

We began this book by talking about the increase in the standard of competition in sport at both national and international levels. There has been a dramatic rise in the number of viable competitors. Sport has become big business, with star athletes and coaches making incredible salaries. All this serves to heighten the pressure that exists in competitive environments.

As the differences in the technical and tactical skill levels of athletes decrease and pressure increases, the role that psychological variables play in determining who wins and who loses continues to grow. For this reason, we will see an increasing demand for the use of psychological assessment in sport. The future is bright. Yet the relative lack of insight into the art and the science of psychological assessment, combined with rapidly advancing technological developments, causes us considerable concern for the future.

In this chapter, we want to share with you our excitement and enthusiasm for what lies ahead. We also want to share our concerns. The best way to begin this process is to briefly summarize some of the critical factors we have discussed in this book:

- Psychological assessment is both an art and a science.

- Validity and reliability as applied to tests are statistical concepts, not absolutes.

- The process of consensual validation is the key to improving accuracy.

Psychological Assessment as both Art and Science

The science of psychological assessment is the process we engage in when we attempt to develop valid, reliable tools and procedures that measure psychological characteristics and enhance our ability to understand, predict, and control behavior. The art of psychological assessment is the process we engage in as we (a) consensually validate or invalidate findings from tests; (b) integrate our findings with performance-relevant situational, personal, and interpersonal factors unique to the client or setting; (c) communicate findings and their implications in a language the client can understand, giving him or her confidence in what we say; and (d) develop intervention programs based on our findings.

As you've worked through this book and engaged in the process of assessment, you should have begun to recognize the major role art plays in the assessment process. With practice, you have become more skilled and more accurate in your assessments of others, but you have also learned that as good as your skills are, there is always more to learn. The difference between the truly gifted assessor and the person who interprets tests is significant.

Validity and Reliability as Statistical Concepts

We hope that by now you have realized that psychological tests aren't either valid or invalid. Instead, tests that we refer to as "valid" and "reliable" typically improve the accuracy of decisions and behavioral predictions by between 10% and 15%. The validity and reliability coefficients associated with our assessment tools tell us how far our "science" has advanced. Based on the relatively small amount of variance currently accounted for by assessment tools, we have a long way to go. Because assessment tools are far from perfect, the responsibility lies with you, the professional, to insure that the conclusions you draw and the decisions you make are ethically, morally, and legally sound.

The Process of Consensual Validation: The Key to Improving Accuracy

Let's say that after testing an athlete, you predict that he will perform poorly in high-pressure situations. Research on the accuracy of this particular prediction, when it is based on test scores alone, indicates you will be correct 70% of the time. This does not mean that 70% of him will choke and 30% won't; nor does it mean that he will choke 70% of the time. The bottom line is that in making this prediction about an athlete under the conditions described, you will be right 70% of the time and wrong 30% of the time.

Can you afford to be wrong 30% of the time? Your goal is to avoid mistakes entirely. Your goal is to be 100% accurate when you make a decision that has potentially serious economic, personal, social, and emotional consequences for an individual. This is the reason assessment is a process rather than a single event. Consensual validation of findings is the most critical element in the assessment process. The process of consensual validation is, to a large extent, an art. It is the art of becoming aware of, and combining, information from different sources in ways that enable you to improve the accuracy of your predictions.

The Future

Will technological advances be used to help us uncover more of the art of assessment, or will technological advances remove art from the assessment process, retarding growth and diminishing the value of the services we offer?

Technology is changing so rapidly that undoubtedly some of the things we write today will be outdated by the time this book is published. Especially in the areas of communication and data management, our world is being turned upside down. Within the last few years, we have seen a breakdown in global boundaries. Today, within seconds, we can have access to people and information from any other place in the world. Let's look at how the breakdown in global boundaries and the ability to manage incredible amounts of data are already having an impact on research, education, and practice in the field of sport psychology.

Technology and Research: The Promise

Today, we have access to a huge pool of data that has been collected on TAIS at Olympic training sites around the world. In fact, at a recent Conference for the Advancement of Applied Sport Psychology (AAASP), we sat in a meeting room and accessed TAIS data from over 10,000 elite-level athletes from Australia, Canada, Italy, Brazil, Spain, France, Germany, and the United States. From that group of athletes, we identified 239 who had won an Olympic medal and/or a world championship. On a computer, we were able to analyze the TAIS data of these medal winners, breaking them into two groups: single-medal winners versus multiple-medal winners. The analysis of that data only took us about 2 hours (Nideffer, Bond, Cei & Manili, 1999).

The opportunities for collaborative research, and for the accumulation of large enough sample sizes to examine highly homogeneous subject groups, are phenomenal. Add to this the fact that the power of today's computers means we can finally begin to develop the complex research designs that will allow us to ask much more meaningful questions, and you will begin to sense some of the excitement researchers are feeling.

Consider these predictions for the future made by Schutz and Gessaroli (1993) in "Use, Misuse, and Disuse of Psychometrics in Sport Psychology Research":

> Technological advances are going to lead us (perhaps force us) into a completely new way of generating and analyzing problems, maybe even into a new way of thinking. . . .

> This interactive hypermedia computer system will enable us to examine complex interactions involving facts and theories, past and present, generalities and uniqueness, all within a common framework. . . .

> Unfortunately, we have not had the education or training to be able even to think about analyses at the level of complexification that will eventually be required. (p. 915)

Technology and Education: The Promise

At the present time, technology enables us to videoconference with instructors in real time—see the instructor, listen to his or her lecture, watch a slide-show presentation, ask questions, etc. The instructor can give assignments to visit the library, and the library may be in Moscow or in London. You may be asked to interview a famous person, and you can locate that person and communicate with him or her, no matter where that individual is. You can go to the Internet and, within a few minutes, locate more resource material than you ever dreamed of. The amount and variety of information available to you are absolutely mind-boggling.

Many of you are probably already involved in taking or teaching courses online. We offer an online course on psychological assessment in sport. We have students in Japan, Singapore, and Europe taking that course. Today, students can have access to the best faculty in the world; campuses are losing their geographical boundaries. At the present time, the primary limitation to online education is the size of the pipeline at the student's end.

Currently, the modems to which individuals have access, the processing speeds of their computers, and the storage space they have available limit their ability to access some highly complex graphics and video information. Such limitations shrink the information pipeline at the user's end. With broadband access, the reduction in computing costs, and the advances that are occurring in the development of faster processors, those handicaps will disappear for many middle-income families by the time this book is published.

Technology and Service: The Promise

As service providers in the field of sport psychology, we deal with clients who are on the road a great deal of the time. Our ability to travel with them is often limited in terms of both the actual time we have available and our ability to economically justify it. Email has made it very easy for us to stay in contact with clients, whether they are in Europe, Asia, or the Americas. They can go online, send us a question, and have a response within minutes. We can chat online, and we can do it for the price of a local phone call.

Today, you can go to the Enhanced Performance Systems website (www.enhanced-performance.com), and if you have been trained to use TAIS, you can have your clients take the inventory online. You, as the trained service provider, will then receive instantly by email a test profile and an extensive psychological report (20+ pages) detailing the individual's concentration and interpersonal strengths and relative weaknesses and offering suggestions for performance enhancement.

Athletes searching for information about sport psychology can go to the Enhanced Performance Systems website and read articles on topics of interest and, if they choose, take an educational version of TAIS, called A.C.E.—Athlete's Competitive Edge.[1] The feedback they receive online from A.C.E. is extensive, teaching them about the arousal, concentration, and performance relationship; helping to sensitize them to their concentration skills and interpersonal characteristics; and offering suggestions for performance enhancement within a sport context.

With increasing frequency, we are finding ourselves involved in consultations on the telephone or via email with professionals around the world. We ask questions to help them target our suggestions and get them to ask questions of their athlete(s) and to observe behaviors that will help them in the consensual validatation of TAIS results. As the communication pipeline (bandwidth) expands, the amount of information we can share and integrate will increase dramatically.

Technology and the Challenges We Face

We've talked about some of the benefits of change and some of the promises for the future, but what about the challenges sport psychology professionals will face? For a long time, the fields of education and the helping professions have been thought of as services rather than as businesses. With advances in technology, however, this is changing dramatically. Education, like sport, is becoming big business, and there is tremendous competition for students. This competition will increase as geographical boundaries continue to break down. The same is true in the helping professions: read the papers and to listen to the concerns that professionals and laypersons alike have about the directions health care is taking.

Until now, educational institutions and the helping professions have been able to rely on geographical boundaries and on legislation to help them protect their particular areas of expertise. Helping professionals have been licensed by states and countries. Licensure laws have served multiple purposes. They have ensured that local, state, and national governments would receive their share of revenues from professionals. They have restricted competition for services, protecting the incomes of professionals within particular geographical regions. They have helped to protect the public by ensuring that individuals offering services meet an identifiable set of standards. These protections are disappearing rapidly. Consider the following:

- A search of the World Wide Web to identify individuals and organizations providing sport psychology services including assessment identified several thousand sites.

- A rough sampling of those sites gave the impression that the professional competency of the individual/organization providing the service was inversely proportional to the attractiveness and packaging of the website. Individuals with excellent computer skills but very little formal training or experience in sport psychology were developing the most appealing sites.

- There were high school students who were selling sport psychology products and services on the Web.

- There were assessment providers offering totally automated assessment programs for selection and screening. In other words, an individual would sit in front of a computer and answer questions. Based on the individual's responses, a decision would be made to accept or reject the individual. The art of assessment had been removed, and we can tell you that the science of assessment has not advanced to the point to justify this type of process.

- From a research perspective, individuals were using the Web to collect data on instruments they were developing. They were analyzing the data and drawing conclusions about the usefulness of the inventories without having the faintest idea as to the identity or the motivations of the people responding to their instruments.

Right now, anybody in the world can claim to be a sport psychology researcher, educator, or practitioner. Right now, anyone in the world, independent of background and training, can promote and sell his or her particular version of sport psychology services and products anywhere in the world. A little knowledge about statistics and Web design, and you are in business. You can create your own assessment tools, and you can sell them.

We have two very specific concerns about the future that we feel must be addressed in order for the profession to survive and advance. The first involves finding ways to educate and protect the consumers of our products and services. The second involves making sure that as professionals, we do not lose sight of the importance of art in the assessment and intervention process.

Protecting the Consumer

To date, we have been unable to reach any kind of agreement at a professional level as to the specific set of core classes and experiences that should be required for practitioners in the field of sport psychology. As a result, clinical psychologists with absolutely no training in the sport sciences, and with very little experience in sport, are calling themselves sport psychologists. There are highly skilled practitioners with a wealth of experience in both psychology and the sport sciences who are restricted to calling themselves "certified sport consultants." Unfortunately, there are also individuals who lack experience in either psychology or the sport sciences referring to themselves as "sports consultants," "performance counselors," "sports scientists," "head doctors," and just about everything else imaginable. This is all very confusing to an uneducated public, a public that too often believes what it reads in the paper or sees on the Internet, a public that is impressed by packaging and wants to believe in magical solutions to difficult problems.

The issue of protecting the consumer is not unique to sport psychology; all of the helping professions must address this. Think of the challenges to be faced here: Which licensure laws apply when someone offers services over the Internet? How can current licensure laws be enforced? True, professions can censure their members or take away their membership, or do both. States can revoke licenses, but so what? How will that prevent people from promoting themselves beyond the state's jurisdiction?

The helping professions have always been seen as a bit exclusionary; many people believe the members of these professions to be as invested in protecting themselves and their territory as they are in protecting the consumer. With the increased competition and opportunity that advancing technology affords professionals, service providers are really feeling the pressure. That pressure is altering focus in both positive and negative ways. On the positive side, it is causing some to evaluate more carefully the services they provide; this is leading to improvements in quality. For others, the pressure is having the opposite, negative effect. Many professionals are paying more attention to packaging than they are to content. Those who are involved politically are scrambling to find more ways to protect their current practices and to expand their opportunities by invading other areas (e.g., the movement of clinical psychologists into the fields of sport, health, and organizational psychology and into medicine and the prescription of drugs). Under the conditions we have described, it is difficult for consumers to make informed choices.

Paradigm Clash

Human beings are caught in the middle of the kind of paradigm shift described by Thomas Kuhn in his book *The Structure of Scientific Revolutions*

(1996). Everything, from who people are to what they do, is under attack. The structures that people have used in the past to organize their world and to give them a feeling of predictability and control are being torn apart. At this point, no one knows what the new structure will look like; no one knows who will be in control.

The information superhighway has created a crisis. Human beings are caught in a titanic struggle between a moral value and principle (the belief that everyone should have open access to information) on the one hand and a basic survival need (the need for structure and predictability in a highly complex world) on the other. At some point, the need for structure and direction will win the battle. Right now, however, no one knows how long that will take or what the future will look like when it happens—and that's frightening.

A look at the business world reveals several important trends. Companies are merging, for a couple of reasons. One reason is to develop and control huge databases—databases that include everything from old films to scientific data. The second reason is to control the information pipeline, how people access it, and what flows through it.

This trend is not limited to private corporations. Governments are getting involved. A recent article in the *APA Monitor* indicated that the National Science Foundation would be making research grants contingent upon the researchers' opening up their databases to others. At the same time, organizations and national groups are creating intranets that limit access to information. Concerns over privacy further push for censorship and limited access to information.

At the present time, there may be a few countries that are so poor and/ or so authoritarian that they are capable of limiting access to information and of remaining relatively isolated from the rest of the world. That will not last long, and as those boundaries break down, people will find themselves subjected to a "new world order" (to borrow a phrase). Will that new world order represent your interests and mine? Will it represent the interests of a few global companies? Will your ability to practice in your chosen field be enhanced or restricted? What can you do to prepare for the new structure and leadership that will be imposed? How should you behave between now and then?

Protecting the Art of Assessment

Developing online assessment capabilities and online assessment courses has really sensitized us to the art of assessment and to the danger that rapidly developing technology poses for that art. If you were to examine the programs promoting online education and the promise of the Internet, you would find that at least 99% of the papers, talks, and symposia being presented focus on the technology and on the excitement the technology generates.

The use of technology for technology's sake can be extremely seductive, especially for individuals who are technologically focused to begin with. Too often, the student and the student's needs are ignored or lost in our attempts to develop online courses. It isn't enough to provide individuals with access to information; we have to teach them how to use the information in responsible ways. Yes, technology makes it very easy for us to expose people to information, but do we know how that information is being interpreted and used?

We have emphasized the nature of the relationship between the assessor—the individual administering and interpreting test information—and the client. We have pointed out how important it is that the person responsible for the assessment process be sensitive to situational variables and to all kinds of verbal and nonverbal behaviors. We have argued for the need to develop the skills that allow you to make observations; to generate testable hypotheses; and to then test and refine those hypotheses, finally using them to zero in on an issue and its solution. This is the process of consensual validation.

As teachers, researchers, or service providers who interact with you face-to-face, we can see your responses to what we say. We can hear the tone of your voice. We can see and, at times, feel the tension in your body. In your presence, we become more aware of the situation, more sensitive to the stimuli that are influencing you. When we are there, we don't have to rely completely on what you tell us.

On the other hand, an instructor of an online assessment course may be able to evaluate your ability to assimilate the factual information or content that you are given (though how can we be sure that it's really you who is taking the class?). With current limitations in the communications pipeline, however, that instructor's ability to observe you in action is extremely limited. How does that individual know that you read the situation correctly if he or she is not there? How does the instructor know whether you paid attention to the right things? How does he or she know the response set that you created for the client? After all, the client's response set is influenced not only by what you say but also by how you say it, by who you are, and by a hundred other situational variables that may be operating. How does your online instructor know whether you communicated your findings accurately and clearly to the client?

Our ability to consensually validate information is as much an art as it is a science. Our ability to inspire clients to have confidence in us and in the things we say, along with our ability to motivate them, is as much art as it is science. Science without art is blind and insensitive. Art without science is superstition. The art of assessment is the science of assessment that has yet to be defined. By observing the artists in our field and identifying the reliable conditions upon which their insights are based, we advance our science. As our art leads to the generation of hypotheses and the development of theories that increase our ability to understand, predict, and control behavior, we transform a portion of our art into science. We make that part of our art operational and teachable.

Currently, many parts of the assessment process remain artistic and cannot be taught in any systematic way. We talk about "intuition" and "instinct," about processes like "learning to listen with the third ear." As an athlete recognizes when he or she has entered the zone, we recognize intuition and insight when they occur in ourselves and in others, but we do not really know why they occur, and we have not learned to teach them or to produce them on demand.

To advance the science of assessment, we not only need to identify new and better measures of existing constructs, but we also need to transform as much of the art of assessment as we can into science. Just as there are athletes who have wonderful physical gifts, so, too, are there practitioners who are gifted with insight and intuition. We should be studying these individuals to discover what it is about their life experiences, about the hardwiring of their brains, about the specific things they attend to, and about the ways they acquire and process information that allows them to see connections between events, and solutions to issues, that the rest of us fail to see. As far as we know, very little of this type of research is being done.

At this point in time, we can program the science of assessment into the computer, but we can't program the art of assessment into it. We can't program the computer to do something that we don't understand. We can't program the computer to do something for which we are unable to create explicit and consistent rules. Because sport is big business, and because the science of assessment is much easier to understand than is the art of assessment, there are some consumers who could not care less about the art—consumers who want to simplify their decisions and their lives; consumers who want tests, consultants, and assessment processes to make decisions for them. Because professionals are in competition, there are people out there who will give these consumers what they want and will claim to be providing better service, because their approach is "more scientific."

You Are the Future

The future of the field is, to some extent, in your hands—perhaps more than you realize. We have confidence that down the road, structures will be put into place that will define the field in a way that protects consumers. At this time, we do not have any reason to believe that currently established professional associations will make those decisions.

Control over technology will not be left to professional organizations. Control over technology will occur because businesses and governments need to protect their investments and their citizens. When the structure is imposed, to whom will that governing body listen? One person might make a decision based on personal experience or friendship; that's certainly happened before. A committee might be formed to try to have various organizations and groups reach some kind of consensus. A panel of experts might be identified to create a structure.

It is our behavior as individuals, as professionals, and as organizations that will determine how the field will be seen and how it will be restructured as the dust settles. It is how we behave between now and then that is critical. We believe that it is to our personal advantage, to the advantage of our profession, and to the advantage of the end users of our services for us to place the needs of our clients and of our field above our own immediate needs.

You have gained some valuable skills, skills that you can use to help others and to advance the science of sport psychology and assessment. To do so, you must be sensitive to both the science and the art that are involved in everything you do as a professional. Twenty years from now, the world will be profoundly changed, and so will the roles and functions of sport psychologists. By that time, members of our profession will have uncovered many of the secrets to the art of assessment and practice, but they will never uncover them all. It is up to you to continue to find and nurture both the scientist and the artist in yourself and in those you hope to serve.

Suggested Readings

Kuhn, T. S. (1996). *The structure of scientific revolutions.* Chicago: University of Chicago Press.

Nideffer, R. M. (1998). *Trading an I for an eye* (Online). San Diego: Enhanced Performance Systems. Available: http://enhanced-performance.com/nideffer/articles/articles.html

Nideffer, R. M., Bond, J., Cei, A., & Manili, A. (1999). *Building a psychological profile of Olympic medalists and world champions* (Online). San Diego: Enhanced Performance Systems. Available: http://www.enhanced-performance.com/nideffer/articles/articles.html

Schutz, R.W., & Gessaroli, M. E. (1993). Use, misuse, and disuse of psychometrics in sport psychology research. In R. N. Singer, M. Murphey, & L. K. Tennant (Eds.), *Handbook of research on sport psychology* (pp.901–917). New York: Macmillan.

Index

N

R

About the Authors

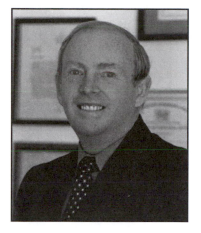

Robert M. Nideffer received his PhD in clinical psychology from Vanderbilt University in 1971. A former associate professor at the University of Rochester and professor at the California School of Professional Psychology, he is currently an adjunct professor at San Diego State University. Dr. Nideffer is the author of 15 books and over 100 articles related to assessment and performance enhancement. He is the founder and CEO of Enhanced Performance Systems, a company that develops and provides performance enhancement products and services to elite level performers and organizations around the world. He has been the sport psychologist for several Olympic teams and has been recognized by his peers as a world leader in the field of sport psychology. You can learn more about Dr. Nideffer, his company, and his work by going to *www.enhanced-performance.com*.

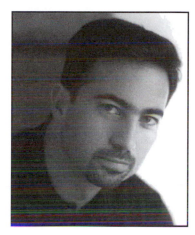

Marc Sagal is Chief Operating Officer of Enhanced Performance Systems (EPS). He has consulted with Olympic and professional athletes from around the world and has conducted psychological assessment and training for fortune 500 companies. Marc has developed a new model of the structural features of competitive sport based upon his research and work with high-level performers. He has authored publications relating to both theoretical and practical issues in performance psychology and has presented research data and professional papers at prestigious international congresses.

A Phi Beta Kappa Philosophy graduate from The Colorado College, Marc received his masters degree in sport psychology from San Diego State University where he was selected as the Outstanding Graduate in his class. Marc holds a United States Soccer Federation "A" level-coaching license and has played professional soccer in the United States, Belgium, and Sweden. He has represented the United States in several International competitions. Marc resides in San Diego, California.